D1621901

PAIN IN THE OFFERING
Hoping and Coping in a World of Hurt

Terry Michaels

Foreword by Charlotte H. Smith M.D.

Edited by Birdie

All scripture quotations are from the
King James Version of the Bible.

Cover image provided by istockphoto

Table of Contents

Foreword

Finding a cure for chronic pain remains one of the most elusive challenges faced in modern medicine.

In over 20 years of practicing medicine as a Physical Medicine and Rehabilitation physician, I've seen and cared for patients with a wide variety of conditions causing chronic pain. In treating persons with spinal cord injuries, brain injuries, neurological conditions, musculoskeletal injuries, back injuries, amputations and other diagnoses, it is devastating to see pain resulting in functional compromise. Often times, the pain is a bigger limiting factor than the paralysis, amputation or other impairments caused by the medical condition. It sometimes completely incapacitates patients and adversely impacts their families and loved ones.

Despite advances in diagnostics, interventional procedures, medications and surgical procedures, many patients fail to find relief. Without solutions from healthcare providers, many give up and lose hope. Often times, prescribed treatments such as surgery or pain medications can actually make the problems worse, resulting in addiction, side effects or other medical complications. As a physician, it can be overwhelming to care for such patients when there are no easy answers or solutions for their pain.

Clearly, there are other factors contributing to chronic pain that we cannot measure or fully understand. We are only beginning to appreciate the role that physical, emotional or psychological trauma plays in the perpetuation of pain cycles. A more mysterious aspect of pain is the role that spiritual factors play in the development and resolution of pain. These spiritual aspects are often either ignored completely or exploited in vulnerable patients. Because there is tremendous potential in this arena, this is tragic.

Pastor Terry Michaels is unique in his understanding of the spiritual aspects of chronic pain. As a Bible scholar and highly effective teacher who has experienced chronic pain, he is able to bring clarity to some of the issues related to this condition. His transparent sharing of his journey, reveals many of the truths that I've also discovered in my medical practice. There is emerging medical evidence that there is a strong neurophysiological basis to support many of his insights. Understanding the spiritual struggles and having strategies to defeat spiritual warfare may provide a missing link for many seeking a cure.

This book will provide encouragement and hope to those who struggle with chronic pain.

Charlotte H. Smith M.D.

INTRODUCTION

SUDAN

Sudan. I wouldn't say I'd never go again. Actually, I'd love to. Only next time I won't go alone. It was a rough trip. A good trip, but rough nonetheless. I was recently invited back. My heart screamed, "Yes!" My body yelled, "No! No more planes or trains or automobiles! No more long trips until you're better! Nothing outside your zip code!" This is my reality now. It's a reality I hate because I like to go places. I'm a full-on missionary at heart. As a pastor, missionary trips do wonders for me. They improve my perspective. They inspire. They build character. They hold promise of vision and needed change. I guess what I'm trying to say is that God uses these mission trips as rescue missions in my own life. He rescues me from the trap of the daily rut and the snare of western ignorance. Somehow, when I see how God moves in other parts of the world I discover how I should be moving in my part of the world. He speaks in strange places unlike He does in familiar surroundings. I can't explain it; He just does.

My trip to the Sudan changed me entirely. I had lost focus and it was in the African bush that I got it back - especially in the area of worship. It was about this time that our growing church relocated. We were a young fellowship and had finally arrived in our own building.

Naturally, this was an exciting time for us. Though we gained a facility, we lost our worship team, at least most of them. We had been scaled down to an acoustical trio: one guitar, a jimbei and a vocalist. They were a talented trio, but it just wasn't what our fellowship had grown accustomed to. Plus our new stage looked as void as a banqueting room set for two. It seemed overkill… and odd. Honestly, this was one of those changes I had not expected with our big move. Nor was I excited about it. I was worried… discouraged… and on my way to Africa.

God found me in the Sudanese village of Nimule. Deep in the bush, in a massive structure of mud, I attended church service. It was a gathering of over 200 people. The room was hot and sticky. There was neither air conditioning, nor electricity to run even a small utility fan. There were no chairs to sink into, just rows of packed dirt that served as pews. There were no lights, stage, sound system, drum set, keyboards or electric guitars. But there was worship! Yes, there was plenty of that! What they lacked in technology they made up for in spirit, and God, true to His Word, inhabited the praises of His people. Their instruments were all handmade. Some shook tin shells filled with pebbles, others rapped their hands against animal skins stretched around circled tree branches. Everyone sang as one, filling the room with a joyful noise unto the Lord.

This style of raw worship may sound primitive to some, but it was not like anything I had ever experienced. It brought me to my knees and reduced me to an emotional wreck. At the risk of sounding like a blubbering baby, I wept. I realize that it's a mistake to measure the genuineness of anything by our feelings. And, trust me, I have preached many times on how deceptive feelings can be, especially when it comes to discerning spiritual matters. But this worship was as real as my tears! Perhaps that is what moved me. I had entered into something so pure and so authentic. No one was there to entertain or impress. They all sang from their hearts to an audience of one.

I suppose I had to be reminded of the kind of worship God desires. He doesn't care about technology. He is not impressed with big stages or bright lights or fancy sound equipment. He doesn't give a rat's whisker about how cool the band looks or how professional they sound. Worship can take place without any of that. I'm not suggesting God is opposed to these things. They're just not necessary. And there is an ever-present danger with them. Just as our feelings can carry us away, so can all the bells and whistles that we rely on to conduct church. It's easy to forget about what is important or what is real. God had to take me half way around the world to remind me of that. He had to free me from my daily rut and remove the veil of western ignorance so that I could see clearly. And in that African bush He assured me that our worship service in small town Texas would not suffer in the least. Stripping our worship team was His way of pruning the dead branches that we might have genuine, vibrant worship – the kind I saw in Sudan.

In a society like America where we are spoiled with technology, toys and an abundance of other frivolous things, we tend to stress and worry a lot. Expectations run high. We also get mad a lot. We may even get mad at God if things don't go our way. We file car problems and computer viruses in the category of Christian suffering. We throw fits over what we think are entitlements. We call ourselves victims when life doesn't go as smoothly as Mr. Lucky-pants next door. I mention these things because stress is no friend to physical pain. Oftentimes, it can be the root cause.

We sometimes joke about people in third world countries because they are so laid back and carefree. They say things like "no problem" or "don't worry, be happy." I would agree that this mindset can be taken to an unhealthy extreme, but I do appreciate the fact that these folks aren't bogged down with all the useless worrying we do in the States. Never did I meet anyone in the Sudan who worried about what to wear or what to eat. They don't stress over things like the light bill or computer crashes. The Sudanese live in a different reality. In this war torn region of the world, people understand what true suffering is. They deal with famine and disease on a daily basis. Or if you're a border town like Nimule, you live with the constant threat of the *Lord's Resistance Army*[*] from Uganda. They come, kill, rape and pillage. They abduct any male child big enough to hold a machinegun.

In Nimule, they don't air TV shows like 'What Not to Wear' or 'The Best Thing I Ever Ate.' They have never

---

[*] Radical military group based in Uganda. They are responsible for widespread murder, rape, abduction and mutilation of African people in Sudan and the Congo.

even seen the *Food Network*. If they did, a popular program might be 'The Only Thing I Ever Ate.' Beans and rice is pretty much it for most. And many Sudanese aren't so lucky to have that. The expression "three squares" is not something you'd ever hear in places like Nimule. Life is simple. Expectations never venture past the unreasonable. The Sudanese would never dream of the silly demands we often place on God. Yet they see miracles we never see. Daily survival is considered a miracle for those in the African bush. It's a miracle for us as well. They just happen to realize it. We don't. We think life is unfair when we don't have our things. We've become prisoners to them.

I did happen to visit some prisoners in the bush. These were real prisoners - prisoners of war! These radical Muslims had been captured after a brutal attack on Nimule. They were the ones who came to kill, maim, rape and pillage. These were the few who didn't get away. There were about sixteen of these captives in total. I had the opportunity to share the gospel with them. I kept it simple. I explained to them of how they could know God and have the assurance of salvation. The Qur'an teaches otherwise, so I knew this would have great appeal. I read to them from *John* chapters one and three. When I asked if anyone would like to give their lives to Jesus, twelve raised their hands. We gave them Bibles in their Arabic language. When our team left, they asked if we could come back and share more Scripture about Jesus.

This was a momentous day for me. My heart was filled with rejoicing and my eyes flooded with tears. *Souls had been saved! Jesus had set the captives free! Hooray!* I was buzzed for hours. But once I came down from my high I got curious. I couldn't help but wonder what these prisoners had actually been deprived of. How had their lives become any different, or any worse than the average African? The only thing that popped to mind was family. Other than that, what did they have to go back to besides a machinegun? It makes you wonder who the real prisoners in our world are. Far too many are prisoners to things. Stuff keeps us in bondage. We are slaves to our entitlements. At the threat of losing things, we worry, we stress and we get mad. We may even get mad at God, even though He warns us not to let material things rule our lives.

I fell in love with the people of Nimule. Even though they have few things and live in constant threat of danger, they seem very content with the hand that has been dealt to them. They don't complain. They don't expect better. They are not angry with God for what they lack. They worship Him. They worship like I've never seen people worship. God spoke to me in the Sudan. In a course of two weeks, He changed my heart, adjusted my attitude and opened my eyes. I returned to America a different person. Spiritually speaking, I was changed. I had changed physically as well. Shortly after my trip I was introduced to the reality of pain. Excruciating pain. Why? How? What? Was it a parasite that I had brought back from the bush? Disease? Cancer? All I knew was that something was wrong - painfully wrong. I hurt something fierce. Six years later, I'm still fighting the pain. At least I'm still in the fight. I refuse to be taken prisoner.

Chapter 1

When I Dream

Dreams really do come true. I've seen it happen on TV. I've watched people become the next iron chef, top model and ultimate fighter. I once witnessed some lucky guy win his very own bachelorette. I even saw a complete unknown become an American Idol right before my eyes. Then there was the biggest loser that became the biggest winner. I've also watched scores of blue-collar types become instant millionaires. Bless their hearts; they all said wealth would never change their lifestyle.

Typically, when people talk about pursuing a dream, they have their sights on something obtainable - maybe not easily obtainable - but obtainable nonetheless. Sometimes, dreams do fall into a person's lap, as we see on TV. But not everyone can rely on luck. Most of us have to pay dues. Living in the land of opportunity does have its advantages. The American dream makes it much easier for those who are hungry for success, whereas third world countries present challenges we don't face in the states. In many parts of the world, people dream of food on the table. For this reason, many dream of coming to America. They have no ambition of becoming the next rock star, sports star or movie star. All they have on their radar is a more comfortable existence. In this stage of my life, that's all I'm after.

I am absolutely convinced that my dream will come true. One day soon I will wake up completely pain free. I often wonder what that will be like. I have forgotten what it is to feel "normal." I'm not sure what that means anymore. My pain is chronic. It is never absent. A day never goes by - not even a moment - when I'm not aware of my discomfort. It's part of me now; a part of who I am. I prefer not to be thought of this way by others, so I don't talk about my condition much... unless I really have to. I refuse to be pitied or labeled. I don't want to be looked upon as that poor, suffering soul. Yet that is how I have come to know myself. I hurt. Sometimes I hurt a lot. I have bad days and sometimes I have even worse days. I couldn't adequately describe what a good day is for me. I suppose that would be when I don't have really bad days.

On not-so-bad days, when my pain is tolerable, I function pretty well. I can concentrate, be social, be productive and feel happy. I can act as if everything feels normal. But even my not-so-bad-days tend to end early. Eventually I tap out. Evenings are the most difficult. By then, I feel fatigued and sorer than before.

Generally, I have to lie down; I stay that way until I turn in for the night.

Sleep is something I have come to truly cherish. In this tranquil state I become oblivious to pain and snooze like a baby. For this reason, I have grown to appreciate those nights of slumber more than ever before. It's the only time can enjoy the normal life. If only I could wake up to this kind of normal... even for a moment. But that's only a dream. That's okay because I truly do believe in dreams. I know mine will come true. Someday soon I will wake up completely pain free.

I will never stop dreaming this dream. No one can ever take it away from me. I will never stop believing or hoping or praying. These things are what keep me going. They are what keep me strong and encouraged and joyful. That's how I prefer to be known by others. I wish to be seen in a positive light, as one who keeps his spirits high. So I dream my dreams and pray my prayers. And I look forward to that day when I will feel normal again. I may have forgotten what it is like, but I do remember it as being pretty sweet. Once I return to the sweet life, I will be known as the one who never gave up on his dream.

"Forsake me not, O LORD: O my God, be not far from me.
Make haste to help me, O Lord my salvation."
(Psalm 38:21-22)

Chapter 2

This is Your Life

I once met a fellow in Nimule named James. He was blind. He wasn't born that way; he lost his eyesight after an assault. The way James explains it - he couldn't come up with the dowry he owed for his bride so his in-laws came after him and doused his eyes with acid. After blinding the poor fellow, his bride was forced to return home. Such is life in Sudan.

It seems to me that one might be better off being born blind than to have their sight taken away later in life. That would be my preference. The way I see it, it's hard to miss something you've never had in the first place. But once you've seen true beauty, it's a privilege you never wish to surrender. Personally, I don't know how I would cope if I could never see a sunset again, or the sparkle in my wife's eyes when she smiles or butter melting over a stack of hot pancakes. I can't imagine what the four seasons would be like without eyesight, or Thanksgiving or Christmas with all its festive lights and fancy decorations. I'm not prepared to give up the gift of sight. James had no choice.

I'm sure James misses the good old days, when he could look upon those things he deemed as beautiful. I wonder if he can still see them in his dreams, or if his dreaming days are over. Has he forgotten what it is like to just sit and stare and absorb everything within view? Does he remember the beauty of a sunrise or sunset? Does he recall that girl he fell in love with, her face, her smile or the darkness of her skin? Or, after a while, does everything fade to black? Does time steal the sweetness away?

James has no hope of regaining his sight. He does not share my dream of one day being better. He accepts his condition. Blindness is his reality from here on out. Fortunately, not all his hopes have been dashed. James decided to turn tragedy into triumph. Rather than focus on what he cannot do, he concentrates on what he can do. When I met him, he was pursuing his dream to be in ministry. He longs to help others. He wants to open people's eyes to eternal things. These things he can see very well.

There are many like James who must accept their condition as permanent. It's their best shot at rising above the pain. You see, there is strength that comes from knowing. If you know your condition is permanent, you can deal with it accordingly and move forward, like James did. On the other hand, if you know your condition is treatable, you do everything within your power to heal. It's the "not knowing" that cripples a person. It can make one feel rather helpless.

I was once at that place where I did not know. I did not know much about my condition or whether it was temporary or permanent. I did not know whether to seek divine healing or turn to modern medicine. I floundered for a while. I finally sought the help of a doctor. He gave me a painful examination before referring me to a specialist. Then I was referred to another specialist and then another. I endured all kinds of treatments and procedures, but no one had any answers. Soon I began to feel embarrassed. I was convinced everyone thought I was nuts or making things up or merely crying out for attention.

It was about a year later when a friend of mine recommended another specialist. After running a tiny camera into my bladder, he was able to diagnosis my condition. You can't imagine the relief I felt. I was in the recovery room when we received word. My wife, Christy, informed me of the diagnosis the moment I awoke. The news came as a sweet surprise. I was so elated that I literally fell apart, crying for joy. *Finally! Now tell me the cure!* The doctor determined that I had *Interstitial Cystitis*, a painful bladder condition. I was given some pills and put on a strict diet. For six months I gave up caffeine, spices, acidic foods and anything with man-made chemicals in it. I dropped a few pounds, but didn't lose the pain. Neither the pills nor the diet did any ounce of good. That's when I gave the holistic approach a shot. Nada. So I gave up on everything: doctors, diets, pills and herbs. All they offered were false hopes and a fallen countenance.

Eventually, I did what James did. I accepted my condition as permanent. It was a sad moment in my life. I still remember it well. My wife and I were driving to Dallas. Actually, she was driving. With my condition, it is better this way. In the passenger seat I can shift around and stretch a little. This helps alleviate my discomfort somewhat; however this particular trip to Dallas was on one of my not-so-good days. It was then I said to myself, "This is your life now. No one can help you." I wept. I mean I really, really wept. Not because of the pain, mind you. I was mourning the death of a friend - Mr. Normal. I had put him to rest… buried him… then bid farewell to a pain free existence. It really did feel as if I were at a funeral. There was that terrible sense of loss. I was really going to miss the deceased. I would miss him for as long as I lived.

That was then, this is now. Six years later, I'm bent on getting well again. Even on the worst days, I look for light at the end of the tunnel. I dream. I pray for healing. I feel it within reach. It's close. I know it is.

"For he hath not despised nor abhorred the affliction of the afflicted;
neither hath he hid his face from him; but when he cried unto him, he heard."
(Psalm 22:24)

Chapter 3

Moving Forward

An early inspiration of mine was John the Baptist, but not the one you're thinking of. This is another. His name actually was John, but everyone knew him as "The Baptist." I first saw him at church, shortly after I came to the faith. It was the first time I had stepped inside a church in many years. Jeff, a coworker, had taken me there. He had also brought Brian, another party-hearty coworker of ours. Jeff hoped to see him get right with the Lord like I did.

Running a little late, we tiptoed into the sanctuary and sat toward the back. I noticed John right away. He was hard to miss. He was the one in the wheel chair with limbs like pretzel sticks. He couldn't have weighed more than eighty pounds tops. He barely had enough muscle to hold his head upright. I felt real sorry for him.

The preacher did his thing. He preached Jesus and he preached with power and conviction. At the end of his sermon, he invited anyone who needed prayer to come forward. Brian was on his feet quicker than a flea hop.

He was finally ready to make peace with God. Others followed. Then I saw John make his way down the isle. My heart sank. He'd probably been down this road countless times before. I had already played the entire scene out in my head. John would wheel up to the altar, the preacher would lay hands on him, mumble a few words and shout, *"In Jesus name!"* Ultimately, John would roll away utterly disappointed. He might even be put on a guilt trip should he overhear the mindless accusation, "He just didn't have enough faith!"

I must say John gave it all he had to wheel himself to the altar. It took every ounce of energy he could muster. He pulled up right next to Brian. With his remaining strength, he slowly lifted his crippled arm then placed his frail hand on Brian's shoulder. "How can I pray for you?" he inquired. Boy, did I have John pegged all wrong! This guy was a stud!

If anyone appeared to have needed prayer that night, it was John. But John didn't see it that way. He had accepted his condition. He was bent on moving forward. Rather than focusing on himself and his needs, he focused on another and his need. That was a huge lesson for me in my early Christian experience. It still resonates to this day. John not only demonstrated the power of love, but also revealed the secret to victorious Christian living.

It is impossible to move forward when the focus remains on yourself and your own pet needs. One must adapt a higher purpose in life. We must allow God to work His will through us in reaching others, helping others and loving others. We will never overcome hardship unless we do. Self-absorption is bondage and only piles misery upon misery. It will make one useless. Only by pouring into others can we achieve any sense of worth. Without this sense of worth there is no incentive to persevere when life clobbers you. There is no point or purpose. You just exist. You become to community what the tonsils are to the human body. You have no real function. You're just there, in the way as a sore spot, spreading pain to other areas.

I realize this goes against the grain of how the human mind normally functions, but it's a time-tested truth. It's one of the divine laws set forth by the Almighty Himself. Surviving hardship requires an upward focus coupled with sensitivity to those outside your own bubble. Both require an immense amount of concentration. That's what love does. It's what real heroes do. This is where true fulfillment is found.

If I might be so frank, there is nothing to be gained by sulking or obsessing over our sufferings. It doesn't help matters one iota. It only makes things worse. Besides, nobody enjoys pouty people. There is nothing to glean from them. They fail to inspire a single soul. You'll never find me following whiners on *Twitter*. I'd have to take a mood elevator first. Pouty people are just too darned depressing. It is heroes like John who make a real difference in people's lives. Their determination to move forward gives the rest of the world hope. Their ability to rise above adverse circumstances is an inspiration to all. I want to be like John. I need to be like that. Meditating on my own misery gets me nowhere very quickly. I go places when I am focusing upward and outward. I can rise above anything. So can you!

"Walk in love, as Christ also hath loved us, and hath given himself for us an offering and a sacrifice to God for a sweet smelling savour."
(Ephesians 5:2)

Chapter 4

Paralyzed

*"For indeed he was sick nigh unto death: but God had mercy on him;
and not on him only, but on me also, lest I should have sorrow upon sorrow."*
(Philippians 2:27)

All of a sudden Christy's hands and feet became tingly and numb. Her legs felt as if she were dragging weighty anvils. Because she was pregnant at the time, we called Christy's OB/GYN doctor. Dr. Munson saw us immediately before referring Christy directly to neurology. The neurologist, wasting no time, checked her into *Loma Linda University Medical Center*. After a week in ICU, Christy came home in a wheelchair. In that brief span of time she had become paralyzed from the neck down. The diagnosis: *Guillain–Barré syndrome*. More than likely, you've never heard of it. Most haven't. It's extremely rare. Here's the 411:

Guillain–Barré syndrome (GBS) [pronounced ghee-YAN bah-RAY]) is an autoimmune disorder affecting the peripheral nervous system. The syndrome was named after the French physicians Guillain, Barré and Strohl, who were the first to describe it in 1916. It is sometimes called Landry's paralysis, after the French physician who first described a variant of it in 1859. GBS has an incidence of 1 or 2 people per 100,000. It is frequently severe and usually exhibits as an ascending paralysis noted by weakness in the legs that spreads to the upper limbs and the face along with complete loss of deep tendon reflexes. With prompt treatment and supportive care, the majority of patients will regain full functional capacity. However, death may occur if severe pulmonary complications and autonomic nervous system problems are present. Guillain-Barré is one of the leading causes of non-trauma-induced paralysis in the world. [*]

As you might imagine, this was a trying time for my wife. It was trying for me as well. There is nothing more tormenting than watching a loved one suffer. I desperately wanted to help. At the same time I felt

---

[*] Wikipedia

utterly powerless. We both did. Then there was the fear of the unknown. It simply could not be known whether Christy's condition was short term or if we were in it for the long haul.

I'll never forget the morning after she came home from the hospital. I turned on the 'Today Show' and would you believe it? They were actually airing a special segment on GBS! Did I just say *special*? It hardly was for us. The gal they interviewed was restricted to a wheelchair and had been for several years. She showed no signs of ever getting out. This was not an encouraging report, to say the least. Unfortunately, I might have flipped the channel a little too late.

Admittedly, I was the whiny one when Christy battled GBS. I just couldn't bear her pain. If it were possible, I would have traded places with her in a heartbeat. She didn't deserve such misfortune. If anyone did it was this guy – yours truly. I was the screw up, not her. That's exactly how I felt at the time. I was the sinner and she was the saint. She was the one being made to suffer. It didn't make sense to me. I thought God was being unfair.

This was one of those seasons the Lord had us face hand-in-hand together. Sometimes it's best that way. To be perfectly honest, I was bitter at first. I had expected our church to make things easier for us. We had been members for over ten years and had poured in hours of service. In our time of need, I thought people would be lining up outside our door, ready to jump at our every beckoned call. What I really wanted was for everyone else to pick up my slack. Looking back, there were some who did. But because of my poor state of mind, the help received was never enough.

Christy, on the other hand, faced her illness with remarkable grace and courage. Naturally, there were also moments of sorrow. I recall her looking outside the window one afternoon as the gal across the street carried groceries from her car. Christy burst into tears. It was the simple pleasures like these that she missed most - things we often take for granted: walking out to the mailbox, preparing a home cooked meal or baking a tray of Tollhouse cookies. She especially missed holding our daughter, Carly. She missed tucking her into bed at night and helping her get ready for school in the morning.

Would she ever enjoy these simple pleasures again? Would she ever be able to walk on the beach? Or hold an ice cream cone? Or plant flowers in the garden? Would she ever be able to embrace that precious child in her womb? We couldn't know.

Though Christy had her down days, her chin always found its way back up. She never once lost her heavenly focus. If I knew my hand wouldn't get slapped, I'd even pencil her name into the Hebrews 11 "Hall of Faith." Don't misunderstand me, I would never wish for a repeat of this experience; however, the Lord used Christy's condition in radical ways to snap me out of a spiritual stupor. Her steadfastness showed me how shallow and selfish I had become. And her undying love for God grew contagious, soaking into me like tiny sparkles of sunshine. I can honestly say I am a new man today because of her influence on me during this difficult season.

Prior to this whole ordeal, I wasn't the most devoted individual, neither in the home nor my Christian walk. I had grown numb and apathetic. Things had digressed so terribly that the idea of a second child had me deeply concerned. I feared it would only prove me a bigger failure. Frankly, I was flat-lining on the inside. Then God threw the switch and administered shock treatment. He also put me in a place where I was constantly at my wife's side, caring for her night and day. We grew incredibly close as a result. All the while, Christy's persistent faith continued to break apart my fragile cocoon. In time, I emerged with a new set of wings, ready to soar to new heights. The Lord used tragedy to expedite a metamorphosis within me. My faith was made stronger. My heart was made softer. My marriage received healing.

Suffering is not something any sane person should ever pray for, but it is also a terrible thing to waste. There is much to be gained once we allow God to use pain for His pleasure. He can accomplish unimaginable good in our lives and use us in miraculous ways to bless to others. We deny Him this opportunity when we grumble, complain or waste away like victims. No good ever comes out of that. My personal prayer is that God would use my sufferings as He did Christy's.

Fellow sufferer, you also are God's chosen instrument. He has called you to bring hope to a hurting world.

There is no greater witness to the reality of Christ. A life of ease does not require much faith nor is it the best showcase for the great work God longs to do. Suffering proves faith to be real… real to you and to others. The world needs to see this kind of faith. If we are going to make a difference on this planet, we must allow God to show His strength through our weaknesses. We must demonstrate His power through our pain. That is the high and holy purpose of our unique calling. It is not God's intention to trap us in a cocoon. He desires to give us wings to soar with. He longs to be the wind beneath them. He wants us to rise in glory!

* * *

In case you were curious, Christy had a full recovery. By the time our daughter Birdie was born, she was well enough to hold her.

Chapter 5

It's the Little Things

I wanted to be accurate, so I showed Christy the rough draft to the previous chapter about her battle with GBS. The memories were too emotional for her, so she had to put it down before finishing. However, she did review enough for me to make some necessary changes. To my shame, I didn't recall all the precious people from church who came by to show some love. Perhaps the stupor I was in at the time caused a mental block of some sort. It's much like how many from my generation can't remember the sixties. It all blurs into a purple haze. Say, wasn't that a song? I can't remember.

We were sitting at *Starbuck's* sipping lattes when Christy recounted the time some gals came over to clean our house. They had done a real thorough job, too, removing every last spec with a fine-toothed comb. I don't actually remember how spotless they left the place, but because this was such a kind gesture, they deserve the benefit of the doubt. Plus, I need to redeem myself for my forgetfulness and for having been such a jerk back then.

From what I'm told, these feather-dusting friends went well beyond the call of duty in primping up our humble home. They even asked Christy if there was anything else needing to be done. She thought for a moment before pointing to the baseboard of the floor saying, "I feel a little embarrassed about this, but could you remove that itty-bitty sticker?" It was one of those cute kiddy decals like *Strawberry Shortcake* or *My Little Pony*, something a small, playful girl would enjoy. Evidently, it had been there for weeks and had finally morphed from a lovable cartoon character into a fly in the ointment. At least in Christy's mind it had. I'm still trying to remember it.

Had Christy been able to, she would have peeled that thing off the floor in a heartbeat. Instead, the gummy perpetrator taunted her every time she rolled by on her wheelchair, and there was no getting around it. This screwy decal became like one of those irritating tags that come on cushions. You want to rip it off but you know it's illegal and you don't want the pillow patrol busting down your door. I don't understand why Christy never asked me to deal with that annoying culprit. As she recalls, it seemed too petty of a request in light of everything else I was doing for her. No doubt, removing *My Little Pony* from the baseboard would have blown the fairy dust out of my wonderful world of rainbows.

There were others from church that came by to show some love. A few folks brought meals. I'm certain this is no reflection on their cooking, but my memory proved to be fuzzy about this as well. That is until Christy brought it up at *Starbuck's*. She said it was the first time we tried Esther's 'Chinese chicken salad with peas,' which has since become a family favorite. It's been years since Christy prepared this dish, so I'm not entirely responsible for forgetting about it.

One sad thing Christy remembers is that no one thought to pray with her when she had GBS. Well, one individual did. He made a point of ministering to all the gals and eventually caused quite a scandal with his friendly "house calls." This good sport aside, no one else prayed with my dear wife. I'm certain they prayed *for* her. They just didn't pray *with* her. This is something I do remember well. I also remember Christy desiring this. She truly appreciated all the help and the many kind gestures, but she desperately yearned to hear someone cry out to God on her behalf.

We all need prayer warriors in our corner but even they have areas of weakness. Sometimes they neglect the practical. They can't seem to unfold their hands long enough to help those they pray for. Most aren't like that, though. Most are the complete opposite. They busy themselves like *Energizer* rabbits with the practical while prayer unwittingly falls by the wayside. Effective ministry calls for a proper balance of both - each reveals a level of compassion. Coupled together, this dynamic duo goes twice as far. It's ironic how most of us are prone to be like Martha, busying ourselves with the more demanding task of service when prayer is so simple. It's much like removing a sticker from the baseboard. You just have to be willing to get on your knees for a few seconds. And once you rise up, you will have alleviated a whole lot of frustration for someone. This is something we all need to remember.

"Now I beseech you, brethren, for the Lord Jesus Christ's sake, and for the love of the Spirit, that ye strive together with me in your prayers to God for me."
(Romans 15:30)

Chapter 6

Life on the Edge

I have a difficult time imagining all those things John
Lennon sang about in the seventies; however, I do
spend a great deal of time imagining no pain and no
suffering. Now, you may say that I'm a dreamer. Well,
I'm not the only one. There are plenty of us who
imagine a pain free existence. To the rest of the world, I
would suspect this is unimaginable and difficult to
relate to. You really have to suffer a chronic illness to
understand.

On my bad days I dream of better days. On my better
days I dream of perfect days, days of no pain and no
suffering. I want it so badly I can taste it, but I honestly
can't imagine what my frame of mind will be once the
battle is finally over. Now that pain has become such an
intricate part of who I am, will I miss it in some warped
way? Will I know how to function without it? Will I
feel like a missionary returning home? I know that last
question sounds like it came from left field, but follow
me on this one.

When I moved my family to the mission field, we didn't serve under the umbrella of an organization that required we raise x-amount of support. We went with hardly any support at all. Not only that, but I also left a high paying government job with all the perks and benefits. We left family, friends, our church of fifteen years and a comfortable home in the suburbs, all to live in a tiny flat in Siegen, Germany. It's amazing what happens when every prop is kicked out from under you. One quickly realizes that God is all you've got. One also learns that He is all you need.

Prior to the missionary life, faith was something I knew mostly in theory. Faith takes on a whole new meaning when one must rely solely upon the Lord, day to day, for absolutely everything. I confess it was a real challenge for me to trust God to meet our every need. There were times when we didn't know where our next meal would come from or how we would pay rent. But not once did the good Lord ever fail us. Sometimes we were brought to the very edge, but He always came through. This does not mean that trusting Him was never a struggle. It was. My faith was stretched to the max.

Honestly, I miss the struggle. I miss those days of crying out to God and watching Him pull through at the last minute. I miss living on the edge where miracles blow through like a steady wind. I miss the daily dependence and not taking small things for granted. Sometimes I think the comfortable life is overrated. Without struggle, there would be little excitement in our world. There would be nothing to conquer. There would be little opportunity to see God move. We'd all be on our comfortable couches watching cable programs in which ordinary people buy and build and makeover comfortable houses.

Health and wealth have their merits, but they seem to lead to a shallow existence after awhile. They do nothing to build character. They deprive us of the sweetness and depth that can only come from suffering. We need those "beauty for ashes" moments in our lives. We need those "oil for mourning" experiences. We need tragedies that make us cry. If for anything, just to feel the tenderness of God's hand as He wipes away our tears.

It's not easy living with chronic pain. But at this stage, I don't know how easy it will be to live without it. Don't get me wrong; I am absolutely desperate for a healing. That's the track I'm on and I know I'm getting closer each day. But how will I cope once I'm well? Will I miss the struggle? After the oil of joy comes, will God still be as near? Will my prayer time be as intimate once the beauty arrives? Once the tears are gone, will I still feel His hand upon my face? It's quite a dilemma for me. I love the sweetness that comes with suffering; I just can't stand the pain.

> *"The Spirit of the Lord GOD is upon me; because the LORD hath anointed me to preach good tidings unto the meek; he hath sent me to bind up the brokenhearted, to proclaim liberty*

to the captives, and the opening of the prison to them that are bound; to proclaim the acceptable year of the LORD, and the day of vengeance of our God; to comfort all that mourn; to appoint unto them that mourn in Zion, to give unto them beauty for ashes, the oil of joy for mourning, the garment of praise for the spirit of heaviness; that they might be called trees of righteousness, the planting of the LORD,
that he might be glorified."
(Isaiah 61:1-3)

Chapter 7

I Can't Stand Sitting

I did it again. I thought I had given up, but gave it one last try. We were at a pastors/leaders conference in Dallas when it happened. Those that desired prayer for a healing were invited to stand. I stood. It was a surprise to me, too. I thought I had already gotten past that with accepting my condition. But I was in pain. I wanted relief. I was ready for a miracle. So I stood. Folks nearby huddled around for the laying upon of hands. Prayers of faith were lifted. Encouragement was offered. A prophetic word went forth, something about the Lord blessing me in my sitting down and rising up, undoubtedly inspired by Psalm 139:2.

The prayers were a huge comfort, but it was that prophetic utterance that really hit me like a ton of *Tylenol*. When I heard that first blessing, my heart leaped while tears flooded my face with the force of a tsunami. How could she have known? She couldn't have. Yet she proclaimed it as if it were truly a word from the Lord. It was. God was telling me He would bless me in my sitting. Perhaps this might sound silly to some, but to me these are words of hope. They are the reason I believe I will be healed someday soon. You see

- my pain is most prominent in my sitting down. For this reason I do a lot of standing. Unless something drastically changes, this entire book will have been written from an upright position. It hurts too much to sit. The longer I do, the more I hurt. So I spend most of my day vertically. I had a counter built in my office that enables me to stand while I work. I eventually get tired of standing. My legs get sore. But God promised to bless me in my standing up too.

Something happened the following Sunday at church. Another miracle. Charlotte asked Christy if I struggled with pain issues. She apologized for the unsolicited examination, but as a doctor she has a knack for diagnosing people when their posture doesn't line up right. Most wouldn't be able to detect what Charlotte detected, but it was obvious to her that my body wasn't well. She saw it in the way I moved. She saw pain. Christy informed Charlotte about my issue. Charlotte offered to help. She said cases like mine were her specialty. She has had great success in making many people well. I will be another one of her success stories one day... one day soon. I wish I could say I'm counting the days, but its not one I can put on my calendar. I just have to be patient and have hope. Yes, hope upon hope.

Once all my medical records were transferred and reviewed, Christy and I met with Charlotte at her office. She insisted I remove my shirt. Then I was told to relax and not worry about trying to impress her. I turned a bright red and let out a hearty laugh. That's when my well sucked-in gut inflated like a beach ball. After examining my frame she told me she saw a perfect 'S'. She was not referring to a big letter on my chest; that was the shape I was in. My side profile was as swerved as a figure-eight racetrack. When she had me touch my toes, I barely made it past my knees. She had me lay on the table for a *Thompson Test*, which I failed miserably. My body was incredibly stiff and guarded. Charlotte said I was the worst case she had ever seen of this sort. I felt worried… and a little proud. I have always wanted to break some kind of record. Unfortunately, I didn't get a ribbon for this one.

Charlotte diagnosed me with *Myofascial Pain Syndrome*, which is a condition characterized by chronic, and in many cases, severe pain produced by knots in the skeletal tissue. Specifically, I have CPPS (*Chronic Pelvic Pain Syndrome*). To quote Wikipedia, *"Pain can range from mild discomfort to debilitating. Pain may radiate to back and rectum, making sitting difficult."* (That's a kind assessment; sometimes sitting is virtually impossible!) Essentially, every square inch of me has been tied in knots for decades, creating a major Charlie horse in my pelvic floor.

Charlotte said my body was the perfect storm. It was just a matter of time before something went south. To illustrate, suppose you fit the opening of a balloon over a leaky faucet. Slowly over time tension builds, the weight inside grows heavier, the rubber walls stretch thinner and to top everything else off, gravity pronounces its ugly curse. It's only a matter of time before something pops. That's what had happened inside of me - only my problem wasn't water retention.

Doctors describe it another way. Before I explain, make a tight fist. Humor me and just do it. Hold that fist as long as you can. Now imagine holding that fist for an hour… a week… a month… a year… forty years. Obviously, you are going to strain muscles, wreck tendons and ligaments and do all sorts of damage, not just in your hand, but also your arm, shoulder and even up to your neck. So, now you have at least two problems. Firstly, you need to correct the damage. Secondly, and most importantly, you need to loosen up. If you don't, more complications can be expected. That's where I'm at now. I'm going through the tedious process of being loosened up.

There are no quick fixes for my condition. The course of action moves at a slug's pace and a lot of work is required. That's why I say I'm on a journey. I have to undo things along the way. I won't reach my destination until I limber up like Gumby. Charlotte has assigned me to an occupational therapist to help me on this journey. Her name is Debbie. I've been seeing her for several months now. She says I've come a long way. That's why my not-so-good days are often elevated to really bad days. Just as I've been warned, things get worse before they get better. I need to be reminded of this every so often, even though it doesn't always make me feel better on the inside.

Chapter 8

I Cry

It's not suffering that makes me cry - it's the journey. I cry when I'm given hope. I cry when I lose it. I cry at signs of progress. I cry when there are setbacks. I cry when I'm strong. I cry when I'm weak. Some are happy tears, others are sad. I'm pretty sure this is normal, at least in the rollercoaster life of one with chronic pain. Tears grow close like a friend.

Not long ago, I left a staff meeting crying. It was one of my not-so-good days and I was in severe pain. The meeting dragged on at the pace of holiday traffic in Houston, leaving my exit nowhere in sight. I grit my teeth the entire time praying for our prolonged powwow to screech to a halt. My body convulsed like mad on the inside, fighting for any smidgen of relief it could find. It was a losing battle. Before long, my mind turned to absolute mush. I lost all concentration. Nothing anyone said made sense. I might as well have been in a henhouse listening to clucking chickens. Honestly, I felt as a toddler might feel sitting through a calculus class.

There were tons of ideas bouncing around but nothing sank in. I just nodded as if everything were crystal clear. After almost two hours of living Sheol, the meeting finally concluded. My exit was abrupt. "Gotta' go," I huffed. "I'm in excruciating pain." I could feel my lips quiver once those words spilled from my lips.

The tears came the moment I turned away and headed for the door. It was not the pain that made me cry, though I'm sure it didn't help any. More so, I was disappointed that I couldn't do what healthy people do. I was saddened by my limitations. I was upset that I couldn't sit down and engage in a simple conversation. I was bummed most of all because I came off as a weakling to my staff. I would prefer they see me as strong. Generally, I do try to be courageous for others. I would rather people not know of my personal struggles. If by chance they find out, I want a testimony of overcoming them. It is also my desire to be a pillar for other folks to lean on. But that wasn't the impression I had made at the staff meeting. I was caught in a moment of dire weakness. I came off as vulnerable. So I left in tears. Oh, the irony of it all.

I hope you don't think I cry a lot. I actually don't; however, I do cry more than I used to. That's just how it's been ever since I bid farewell to the old me. Life is different now. It's a bit more of a struggle. The ups and downs are more profound and more frequent. I actually feel the bumps in a more traumatic way. The tears somehow bring healing. Each drop is like a tiny painkiller. They have a way of soothing my soul. And God always seems to see my tears. He draws near to wipe them and to make me feel better. I don't mind crying in front of my Lord. I have nothing to hide from Him. He already knows my weaknesses. I've placed them all in His hands. That's where I prefer to keep them, between Him and me.

"They that sow in tears shall reap in joy." (Psalm 126:5)

Chapter 9

Freeze

Charlotte recommended that I read 'A Headache in the Pelvis.' Dr. David Wise Ph.D. and Dr. Rodney Anderson Ph.D. of *Stanford University* wrote this odd titled book. These two geniuses have done extensive research on Chronic Pelvic Pain Syndrome. Together they have broken new ground in understanding this condition and developing a protocol to relieve those who suffer from it. After living with CPPS himself for over twenty years, Dr. Wise was determined to find those answers the medical community lacked. His partner, Dr. Anderson, an urologist, has done extensive research with regard to the physiological mysteries surrounding CPPS. Dr. Wise, with his background in psychology, explored the behavioral aspects that might contribute to this condition. His findings shed light on the real root of the problem for many males. Unless the cause is understood, the best that can be offered is a bandage, which does little to soothe the pain or correct the problem.

In years past, pain pills and surgery were the preferred methods for helping CPPS patients. Neither addresses the real crux of the problem. More often than not, they only camouflage it and in many cases make things worse. To use the tightened fist example again, a pill might relieve the pain temporarily, but does the actual condition change? Or if the nerve to the inflicted area is blocked or released, has the real issue been resolved? Absolutely not! So long as that fist remains balled up, something else is going to snap. For so long the wonderful world of white coats focused more on symptoms than the cause of *CPPS*. That is until Dr. Wise and Dr. Anderson did their groundbreaking research. I'm glad they did.

Those who study human behavior have noted two basic responses to fear: *fight* or *flight*. We either kick or run. We face our fears or flee from them. In recent years, a third response has been considered: *freeze*. There are those who neither fight nor flee when threatened. They become as the proverbial deer in the headlights. They tighten up, pant for dear life and tuck their tails between their legs. Dr. Wise and Dr. Anderson have found this to be the case with the vast majority of patients who suffer from CPPS. The tailbone is perpetually tucked in to protect the vitals.

Research has also revealed that most male patients experienced some major trauma (physical or sexual) to cause them to tighten up. In other words, PTSD (post traumatic stress disorder) plays a significant role in pelvic pain. If these studies are accurate, which I'm certain they are, this is why I've been balled up like a fist for so long. Childhood trauma trained my body to be guarded at all times. Over the decades, my pelvic floor has been subjected to tremendous pressure. This pressure intensifies when I'm caught in the headlights of oncoming stress. My tendency is to freeze. According to Dr. Wise, I need to watch my tail and learn to relax more.

Understanding this helps me immensely with regard to my journey to wellness. Firstly, it shows me that my core problem is treatable without having someone cut into me. It can be conquered through deep therapeutic massage, stretching, relaxation, and stress management. In addition to these things, there is also a lot of cerebral exercise as I reprogram my muscles and nerves to behave in a constructive way. As mentioned earlier, it's a long process. I have at least forty years of bad mojo to unravel, which requires a great deal of discipline and determination on my part. The good news is that if I can fix myself, my pain can also be fixed.

It is not necessary for CPPS patients to revisit the trauma that might have led to their pelvic disorder, especially if they have already been there and done that; however, the intent of this book is to help others overcome pain - both physical and emotional. Therefore, it is pertinent that I tell my story. So, as you join me on my journey to wellness, there will be occasional flashbacks. I need to emphasize from the start, I have already dealt with my horrid history and have been totally healed of the emotional trauma associated with the abuses I suffered as a child. Presently, I am no longer at a place where it serves me to dumpster-dive back in time. I believe in moving forward more than I do psychoanalysis or dwelling in the mire of crappy memories. Trust me when I say that as I recount past experiences, it is not for my own benefit, nor was it recommended I do this as a form of self-therapy. My only goal is to help people. As I share the agony of my long-ago maltreatment there will be no wallowing in sorrow. My greater purpose is to share how one can overcome. For now, suffice it to say that I was messed up for many years. But in Christ I am no longer a victim. I have come through victoriously!

"In the day when I cried thou answeredst me,
and strengthenedst me with strength in my soul."
(Psalm 138:3)

Chapter 10

Ode to Jack and Buttons

It's probably not the manliest thing to do, but I've been thinking lately about cats. Christy and I are the proud owners of a grouchy old feline named Buttons. We have to warn people not to pet her, because she'll slice a person's hand off with one sweep of her nasty claws. She's not that big, but what she lacks in size she makes up for in attitude. I once witnessed Buttons tear into a dog twice her size. On a separate occasion, she attacked the neighbor's Miniature Dobey. The owners yanked the little yapper up by the leash, but Buttons remained in tow with her sharp claws secured to the crying canine's ribs.

There are instances where Buttons does allow herself to be pet, however, it has to be on her terms. She must come to you and give the okay. And she will only allow you to pet her in certain places. She likes to be scratched behind the ears. She also likes to have her back stroked. But if you dare try to pet her on the stomach, there will be blood!

Then there is Jack. He is one of Button's offspring, but you would never know it. He is twice her size. Plus he is approachable and extremely lovable. Unlike his moody mama, this giant Tom can be pet anytime, anywhere. Even with just a look, one can make Jack purr like a diesel truck. The only drawback is, gestures of affection are usually paid back in large doses of drool. Aside from his excessive slobbering, Jack is a very pleasant creature.

Jack had the benefit of being born and raised in a nurturing home. That's why he bonds so well with people. The only touch he knows is a loving one. He has had no bad experiences to relate to. He sees no need to fear or to be guarded. All and all, Jack has been smothered with affection his entire life. Buttons, however, has a tragic past. She was abused and abandoned. Being streetwise she knows firsthand that there are touches that can inflict tremendous amounts of pain. That's why she is so cautious and guarded.

Many, like myself, who suffer from CPPS, relate well with Buttons. Our history dictates that some touches are unpleasant and even harmful. Therefore, we are guarded. This does not mean we don't like to be touched, but it requires a great deal of trust before we allow that to happen. Intimate touching is typically on our terms. Areas known to be pleasure zones are oftentimes caution zones. There may not be any resistance, just indifference. A tender back massage, for example, may not offer the intended comfort. It may prove to be an awkward experience unless the pleasure receptors are given the green light to enjoy themselves.

For some of us, there are places we can't stand to be touched at all. There are fears and misunderstandings that must first be worked through. We need help discerning what is safe and what isn't. Just as Buttons must learn that some touches are intended for good, we need to do the same. This is all key to our wellness, because our only hope for a healing is touch.

"Jesus came and touched them, and said, Arise, and be not afraid."
(Matthew 17:7)

Chapter 11

Breakthrough

I'll never forget my first appointment with Debbie. I knew in part what the role of an occupational therapist was, but didn't exactly understand how I could be helped by one. These folks master at stretching and pulling limbs. Judging by the way I felt, one would have better luck with a marble statue than with me. I was convinced that God had created me to be rigid like a GI Joe doll, not bendable like the rubbery Stretch Armstrong. In order to tie my own shoes I had to pray for a miracle. That's how it was and I learned to live with it. I adapted. It was as normal as coffee with cream, maybe with a hint of hazelnut.

To get to my point, the idea of having somebody bend what shouldn't be bent had me concerned. Obviously, I was a unique case, a total mystery to the uninformed world of occupational therapy, so I would have to enlighten Debbie as to my body's unusual limitations. Added to this was an even greater fear. I didn't want to be touched anywhere near my hurt area. I had prepared a speech for that too. It went something like this,

"Don't go there." As Charlotte's had suggested I do, I took Christy with me. Good thing, too. If I couldn't convince Debbie that I was crafted much like a stiff wooden puppet, my dear wife might pull a few strings.

Upon arrival, we were escorted into a small cubicle. A sweet fragrance filled the room while spa music quietly played in the background. It's not as romantic as it may sound. In the center of the floor stood the dreaded bed where I was to make myself "comfortable." Feeling like Buttons the cat, I reluctantly crawled in. Minutes later, Debbie appeared, all smiles and her face glowing with enthusiasm. She spent the first part of our session putting me at ease and winning my trust. She promised that there would be no invasive treatment. Already I could feel my muscles loosening up. Her assuring words had me calmed in no time. I might have even purred a little.

Debbie soon took note of my chest (and not for reasons that might flatter a man). My upper torso was working overtime, like an oil pump on steroids. In fact, Debbie said I was panting like a frightened animal. She showed me how my stomach should be rising and falling, not my collar bone. I was instructed to take longer, deeper breaths and to make this a daily practice for healthy blood flow.

By our second session, Debbie had already proven that God did not design me as a stiff GI Joe doll. After successfully relaxing my body, she folded me into some sort of *Cirque du Soleil* position. I think the heel of my foot stretched somewhere around my upper back. It didn't even hurt in the slightest. I was in total disbelief. Even Christy watched in awe. It was as if we had witnessed the most glorious miracle ever. Neither of us could control ourselves. Together, we cried a river. I was not the stiffy I had imagined. I'm just insanely guarded – like Buttons. It was an emotional moment. I felt like a blind man who experienced sight for the first time, or a lame man who was made to walk, or a captive who had been set free. I had been in shackles for almost my entire life, locked away, held prisoner by my own self and now the gates were swinging wide open.

Though this was a huge breakthrough, I was hardly healed from the pain. The journey had just begun; however, Debbie was able to convince me that I was treatable. We were merely peeling back the onion layers before getting to the core. A huge amount of dedication would be required on my part as well: daily prayer, breathing exercises, stretching, stretching and more stretching.

These days, I feel a lot less like Buttons and a lot more like Gumby. Maybe I will try out for *Cirque du Soleil.*

"The Spirit of the Lord GOD is upon me; because the LORD hath anointed me to preach good tidings unto the meek; he hath sent me to bind up the brokenhearted, to proclaim liberty to the captives, and the opening of the prison to them that are bound."
(Isaiah 61:1)

Chapter 12

Survival of the Fittest

Back when I was in junior high, P.E. coaches would appoint team captains from among the class and, in turn, those kids would pick the players they wanted on their respective teams. Without fail, I was the one they always fought over. *"You take him!"* demanded captain #1. *"No, you take him!"* fired captain #2. That's right, I was dead last every time. It didn't do a lot for my self esteem either. I avoided sports like cafeteria food. Athletics seemed to bring out my three greatest phobias: the fear of failure, the fear of ridicule and the fear of getting my buttowski kicked. Usually, I would fall prey to all three by the first inning, first quarter, or first whatever.

Rather than subject myself to the inevitable humiliation (and a sore buttowski), I would often ditch. Naturally, I would show up for roll call. But by the time attendance was finished, I was already plotting my great escape.

The other boys headed out to the field while I made like Houdini and disappeared into the locker room. Faster than a speeding bullet I would dress back into my street clothes. As soon as my *Wallabies* were tied I did the impossible by climbing atop the double-decked lockers and slithering out the narrow window slat high atop the wall. It took the skill of MacGyver, which gave me a most amazing sense of thrill and accomplishment that could never be experienced in something as dreary as junior high P.E. class.

Whether we care to admit it or not, there is such thing as 'survival of the fittest' among the human species, especially of the teenaged variety. Don't take me wrong; I'm not a Darwinist by any means, but one thing is for sure - the stronger fare better than the weaker when it comes to athletics and other physical challenges. The stronger are more apt to fight while the weaker are more likely to flee. The weak are also subject to being bullied and beat up. Teachers or other authority figures that feel they have something to prove may even bully weaker kids. Trust me, I know.

In my troubled adolescent years, I was pushed around by all kinds of people, even grownups. My sixth grade teacher, Gruesome Yussom as we called him, would often single me out just to show everyone what a bully he could be. Then there was Mr. Janish who lived across the street. I was sitting on my fence one afternoon when he came over, spit in my face and bloodied my lip with a sucker punch. I was no more than ten years old at the time. When I was fourteen, I was beat up mercilessly by an auto mechanic because I threw an empty soda can onto his lot. He chased me down, wailed on me and finished the job by slamming my head into the asphalt. He actually knocked me out! When I came to, he grabbed me by the scruff of the neck and dragged me all the way back to the can I threw so I could pick it up. I complied. I also came home a bloody mess.

Getting beat up was a normal occurrence in my younger years. Even my older brother took the liberty of pounding my face in regularly. I never held it against him, but I never felt safe with him either. Somehow I knew I wasn't the one he was mad at. He became angry when my father left. He needed a punching bag, so I would simply curl up into a fetal position while he went to town beating the living daylights out of me. It would get brutal at times. On occasion, my mother would call the man next door to pull him off. There were also a few times when she called the police. These experiences along with others, taught me to be guarded at all times. I went through life constantly feeling threatened. I wasn't strong enough to fight back. I knew better than to even try. Only two options remained: flee or freeze.

When it comes to my medical condition, however, I am as determined as a Pit Bull to fight. The way I see it, decades of weakness is what ultimately wrecked me on the inside. All those years of guarding literally tied me up in knots. My pain is a product of my own doing and the only way to undo it is to be strong. I have no shot at wellness should I choose weakness. Plus, I just don't want to be perceived as the pathetic whiner, or the victim, or the sorry, suffering sap. Those who give regular updates on their illnesses perplex even me. Some join social networks for that sole purpose. They post things like, "Another bad day today" or "Feeling worse than ever." *Please!* I have lousy days too, but I don't see the benefit of advertising it. There are none.

Rather than throw up the white flag and act like a victim, I choose to march under the banner of a conqueror. I will not accept defeat. I will not allow pain to win. Obviously, there are things I have a difficult time doing which I must accept (like sitting for extended periods). There are also things I shouldn't do if I want to get well. But I don't dwell on what I *can't* do. I focus on what I *can* do. One of the many things I can do is allow God to use my condition for His glory. I can allow Him to use me to speak hope into the lives of others who suffer. But I can only do these things if I am strong. Should I choose weakness, I accomplish nothing. I help no one. I only make myself feel worse, both emotionally and physically. There is nothing to gain through weakness except added pain. Therefore, I choose to be strong. In this world of suffering, I want to be a MacGyver. I want to make giant leaps and tackle the impossible. You see God has picked me to be on His team. I can't lose with Him. He will see me to the last inning, or last quarter, or last whatever.

"In all these things we are more than conquerors
through him that loved us."
(Romans 8:37)

Chapter 13

JFK

Did you know that President Kennedy was wearing a back brace at the time of his assassination? My guess is, probably not. Of course I was quite little at the time, but I never realized that JFK was in such bad shape the entire time he served as commander in chief. I must have missed that day when they talked about it in history class. Word has it he had all kinds of health problems, chronic pain being one of them. His was brutal! According to an article posted in *The New York Times*[*] on November 17, 2002, he suffered from a bad back, persistent digestive problems and Addison's disease among a host of other issues (pelvic pain not withstanding). Below are but a few excerpts from that report:

---

[*] "In J.F.K. File, Hidden Illness, Pain and Pills" Lawrence K. Altman and Todd S. Purdum

"X-rays and prescription records, show that he took painkillers, anti-anxiety agents, stimulants and sleeping pills, as well as hormones to keep him alive, with extra doses in times of stress."

"By the time of the missile crisis, Kennedy was taking antispasmodics to control colitis; antibiotics for a urinary tract infection; and increased amounts of hydrocortisone and testosterone, along with salt tablets, to control his adrenal insufficiency and boost his energy."

"The records show that Kennedy was hospitalized for back and intestinal ailments in New York and Boston on nine previously undisclosed occasions from 1955 to 1957, when he was a senator from Massachusetts, campaigning unsuccessfully for the 1956 Democratic vice-presidential nomination — and quietly planning his 1960 presidential bid."

"The president had so much pain from three fractured vertebrae from osteoporosis that he could not put a sock or shoe on his left foot unaided, the records reveal. He sometimes reported waking before dawn with severe abdominal cramps."

I suppose what impresses me most about all this is that we didn't hear these things from JFK. These aren't his reports. These are reports of doctor reports from those who report the news. Despite his conglomerate of illnesses, President Kennedy somehow managed to rise above his pain. He didn't get caught up in that pitiful victim mentality. The earlier quoted *New York Times* article also notes:

> *"Yet for all of Kennedy's suffering, the ailments did not incapacitate him... In fact, while Kennedy sometimes complained of grogginess, detailed transcripts of tape-recorded conversations during the Cuban missile crisis in 1962 and other times show the president as lucid and in firm command."*

His philandering aside, JFK is best remembered for greatness. His policies may be argued for years to come, but his strength as an individual cannot be denied. As far as I can tell, there are no accounts of him as being wimpy, whiney or weak. Nor was he ever perceived as such while in office. He sucked it up and pushed forward. He did not lay his personal burdens on the nation. Rather, he stepped up to carry the nation's burdens. Perhaps that's to be expected from one who preached, *"Ask not what your country can do for you, but what you can do for your country."*

I once had a friend who served as pastor of a small, struggling church. Bless his heart; he was a very sickly individual. It took everything he had just to show up on Sunday mornings and I give him props for that. When behind the pulpit he proclaimed glad news, but off the pulpit it was always sad news. This dear brother spent endless hours lamenting of all his many ailments. He also had high expectations of the church to take care of him. His needs took first priority and became a huge drain on the tiny congregation. I did feel extremely bad for my friend's condition, but his illness paved way for an unusually lopsided ministry. A pastor is to take the burden of the church and not the other way around. Sadly, my friend missed the opportunity to inspire others.

You may not have the responsibility of minding a flock, but we all have an important job to do. Each of us has a unique calling upon our lives and we must rise up. We were created to be productive and to make some positive contribution to the world around us. No doubt, there are limitations imposed by chronic illness and pain. Some of us may even require special care. But who doesn't have limitations? Each of us must know what they are and gracefully accept them. However, our limitations do not detract from the unlimited possibilities that exist when our lives are placed in the hand of an Almighty God. Consider Joseph. The Book of Hebrews tells us:

> *"By faith Jacob, when he was a dying,*
> *blessed both the sons of Joseph; and*

worshipped, leaning upon the top of his staff." (Hebrews 11:21)

I suppose it's true, it's hard to keep a good man down. Old decrepit Jacob had one foot in the grave and the other on a banana peel, yet he mustered enough strength to rise up. He rose up to bless his sons. He also rose to worship his God. I can't imagine it was easy for him, yet he did it, all because he was willing to rise up. That's all it really takes to succeed in life or to make a difference in the world. All one must do is rise to the occasion. We must rise above adverse circumstances. We must rise above opposition. We must rise above pain and suffering. We must rise even when our bodies say differently.

Chapter 14

They Got My Back

I had to correct a false report from spreading in our church recently. It wasn't anything too serious; it just wasn't accurate. The buzz had to do with me. People were saying I have a bad back. I don't, but I understand why some might think this. It's a natural assumption when you hear that someone suffers chronic pain and aren't given precise details. When folks informed me they were praying for my back, I really didn't know how to respond. Deep down, I wanted to clear up the confusion, but I just don't like discussing my condition. Frankly, I get a little embarrassed pinpointing where I hurt. Does anyone really need to know? Besides, what's the harm with people covering my back? Perhaps I would ache there too if it weren't for the many petitions lifted on my behalf. So rather than set the record straight, I simply thanked those precious saints who were praying for me. Anyway, I'm sure God wasn't confused by the anatomical mix-up.

There are several reasons I keep my issue under a tight lid. The main reason being, I don't want pity. Another reason is that I've had my fill of complementary diagnosis and could use a break from it all. As a pastor of a fairly large church, I run the risk of being diagnosed by a lot of folks who believe this to be their spiritual gift. I used to serve at a much smaller fellowship back when my pain first started. We were gathered for a special night of prayer when I went "semi-public." It was a small group, so I felt safe. News travels fast. Before long, a holy host of bleeding hearts crawled out of the woodwork to offer their analysis. First, they wanted details, which I wasn't so eager to cough up. Even with my cryptic explanation, their remedies were sure as church service on a Sunday morning.

"Try this goop I get online!"

"See Sally at *The Whole Earth Shoppe* and buy some herbs!"

"Try this!"

"Try that!"

"Try *Amway*! Lucky for you, I'm a distributor!"

After being bombarded with a horde of cures and causes, my head was left spinning. I couldn't help but wonder why the experts didn't have answers while everyone else did. I don't fault these dear people. Everybody had his or her heart in the right place. It's just not what I needed at the time, or wanted. All I really asked for was prayer from a few folks.

Coming to a larger church, I was a little more careful, too careful perhaps. Now everyone and their uncle thinks I have back problems. On the upside, no one has offered magical potions, folk remedies or *Amway* products. They have only offered prayer, which I like; however, I did have to set the record straight recently. A couple informed me the other Sunday, "Our home group prays for your back every week." This made me both happy and sad. I was happy that these folks truly cared about me, but I was saddened because they were lifting prayers I didn't necessarily need. So, for the first time, I felt a sense of obligation to clarify my condition. I didn't give a lot of detail, just enough. It really wasn't as horrifying as I had anticipated. And I'm pretty sure that those precious people still have my back.

"I thank my God, making mention of thee always in my prayers;
hearing of thy love and faith, which thou hast toward the Lord Jesus,
and toward all saints."
(Philemon 1:4-5)

Chapter 15

Ringside

One thing I have purposed not to do in this book is come off as whiney. Above all, my desire is to encourage. That said, I ask that you indulge me just this once. There will be a little whimpering in this chapter. You see, I really wanted to go to the fights last night. I had VIP passes, ringside seating and the whole nine yards. Let's just say, I know a guy. He happens to be the state commissioner for fighting events. His name is Big Greg. You'd call him that too if you ever saw him. He is a mountain of a man, one that would frighten anyone out of the octagon.

Big Greg said he wanted to bless me for pastor's appreciation month. (Yeah, a lot of people have never heard of it.) I happily accepted his offer. Not just one but two tickets to the MMA[*] bout in San Marcos. A couple close friends who happen to coach had fighters scheduled to compete. So, if it's possible to have sentimental reasons for attending a fight, I had them. I had them all: a man who wanted to bless me as well as two others who would have appreciated my support. Naturally, I also had my own selfish motives for attending. I'm a huge MMA fan.

---

[*] MMA – mixed martial arts

Then it happened. I had one of my debilitating pain flare-ups. Throughout the day I had hoped things might improve. They didn't. Things only got worse. There was no way I would be able to endure the hour drive, three hours of sitting, followed by the long drive home. My pain would only skyrocket. I had no choice but to call Big Greg and inform him of my disappointing news. It is quite humbling to tell a giant named Big Greg that you can't make it to the fights because you have an ouchie; I felt like a total wuss.

It would be unfair to say that pain has wrecked my life, but it has altered it. I can't always do the things I wish to do - even simple things like sitting at *Starbucks* with my beautiful wife. We do go out for coffee; we just don't stay long. On my not-so-good days, our visits are especially brief. Sometimes I'm not able to go at all. Well, I could. It just wouldn't be very fun. Dinner dates, movies or anything that might involve prolonged sitting all depend upon my pain level. Christy will often ask first, having me rate my pain on a scale from one to ten. That number usually determines how we will spend our time together.

Even on my not-so-good days we plan dates. We simply opt for places where we can be on our feet. For example, last night we walked around *World Market*. I bought dark chocolate. She bought something in housewares. Then we went to *Hobby Lobby*. Life is funny that way. I was supposed to be at the fights, but ended up in an arts and crafts store. Naturally, I didn't see anything I wanted. Christy had a women's function coming up, so she loaded her cart with all kinds of goodies. We finished the evening with frozen yogurt. She filled her cup with mango-peach. I went full throttle on the raspberry-pomegranate. Christy recommended we stand outside and eat. She is very considerate that way.

I realize this wasn't one of those dates most would write home about, but I found it to be especially satisfying. I even got over my blues about missing the MMA bout. Maybe I'll even write a song about it. The chorus will go something like this: *better is one day in her courts than thousands ringside.*

I saw Big Greg at church the following Sunday. It was a little awkward initially. I suppose I was feeling a tad insecure. Did he think I had wimped out? Was he offended that I shot his blessing down? Did he feel I had used a poor excuse? These things go through your mind when you deal with chronic pain. At least they do with me. I worry about being misunderstood. I fret about upsetting others when I have to tap out of something. I was prepared to apologize to Big Greg, explain myself and express my regret, but I was never given the opportunity. He charged right after me, wrapped my body into his huge arms and prayed for God to heal me.

"We are bound to thank God always for you, brethren, as it is meet, because that your faith groweth exceedingly, and the charity of every one of you all toward each other aboundeth."
(2 Thessalonians 1:3)

Chapter 16

Relax

Many have the wrong impression when it comes to occupational therapy. Some think I go for a relaxing massage and that I feel as if I'm on cloud nine afterward. The truth is that not everything Debbie does to my body gets filed under the category of relaxing. But that's not why I go see her. I go to *get* well, not *feel* well. That would be the end result once I'm better, but with my unique condition, the rehabilitation is remarkably slow. And until I am fully rehabilitated, Debbie must do things that boot me way out of my comfort zone. She massages deeply into my muscle, applying the pressure one might expect from a steamroller. It takes everything I have to convince my body to relax. If I don't relax, progress will be hindered. In other words, my chances of improving are about as likely as Eminem going on tour with Manilow.

Relaxation is a whole new discipline for me. My body has been on pins and needles for practically my entire life, so I have to unlearn all those bad habits that make me tighten up. I need to teach my body to just chill. A lot of this comes from awareness. I need to be more in tune with my body to know when it's tense and what makes it that way. I must also tune in once my body gets into a relaxed state and remember what that feels like. I think I now know this better, whereas before that was unexplored territory. I actually thought I was normal prior to seeing Debbie. Seriously, I never realized how balled up I had been until being properly introduced to this thing called relaxation. Then I became like a kid who discovered chocolate for the first time. It tasted good and I wanted more.

Debbie says I've come a long way. In those early sessions, I was about as loose as a tree trunk. That's when Debbie had to say and do certain things to relax me. She taught me techniques I could apply on my own to help calm not just my body but also my mind. I never realized how intricately the two are connected. I suppose I knew this conceptually, but I had mentally disassociated my head from my body as a way of detaching from past trauma. I'll tell you more about that later. The point here is that this relaxation business requires a lot of brainwork, which means I have to get back in touch with myself. It's amazing what I have learned through this process. I have a much better understanding of how God wired the mind, muscles, nerves and emotions to operate in perfect harmony. I have also learned (the hard way) about what happens when they don't. The goal for now is to get things back in sync. My wellness depends on it.

I must admit, after months of therapy I do feel healthier than I ever have before, and I do mean in my entire life. I realize that's a big claim from a guy in his fifties, but it's true. My body is stronger, my nerves are calmer and my mental outlook is also as bright as can be. All and all, I'm extremely optimistic about things. I just hurt in a certain area. But I'm fit for the fight. I will beat this thing before it beats me.

Now that I am healthier and more relaxed, Debbie can focus near the source of where my pain is. Sometimes it feels as if I were in a wrestling match, on the losing end of a submission hold. I have to tell myself not to tap out. It does get a little easier with every visit. The more those muscles loosen up the less I hurt - and the more relaxed I become. I just have to keep reminding myself that not all treatment has to feel good to be therapeutic. It just has to make me well over time.

Chapter 17

Muscle Madness

The last time I saw Debbie she almost made me cry. She pressed on a muscle deep in my pelvis, causing my eyes to well with tears. It wasn't any kind of physical distress that prompted this blubbery reaction. Debbie happened to press into an area known to trigger an emotional response. This is a common phenomenon, one that many massage therapists encounter often. Debbie says there are a host of notions out there as to why this occurs. She wasn't kidding. I have done my own research and it seems there is an ancient theory involving the muscle/emotion relationship that dates back before *ibuprofen* could be purchased at places like *Walgreen's*.

Some suggest that those burdens our minds can't handle are buried in muscle tissue. It's as if our muscles become a hidden hard drive of horror. Bad data is collected there - unless it can be released through a proper expression of emotions. This becomes a problem for trauma victims who can't seem to "let it all out." The data never gets deleted. It gets dumped from the mind to some unsuspecting area of the body. Once full, that storage compartment sends a message in the form of aches and pain. If this theory is correct, that's why I was choking back tears during treatment. Debbie hit on a corrupted file in my storage compartment.

I should point out that not every expert agrees with this theory; however, if I were to use myself as a case study, I'd have to conclude that it makes fairly good sense. Research also indicates that many males who share my rare condition are typically victims of childhood abuse. While it may be difficult to believe that muscle has memory, there is no denying those more scientific studies that identify chronic pelvic pain as a common symptom of post-traumatic stress disorder (PTSD). Things may not flare up immediately after a person experiences distress. That memory can remain calm for a very long period. But as more bad data (stress) piles into the equation, it's only a matter of time before everything comes to a head.

As I said earlier with the balloon analogy, trauma begins when the opening of the balloon is stretched over that leaky spigot. Every drop that falls creates additional stress. The balloon will serve as useful storage for a while, but before long it's going to burst.

Stress is no friend to the body, the mind, or the nervous system. Unless it can be released in a healthy way, something eventually pops. This is why many suffer from headaches, neck aches, backaches and a host of other kinds of aches, not to mention high blood pressure and heart disease. Even if one's pain is the result of an injury, stress can magnify it immensely.

As a troubled youth, I did not handle trauma in a way that could be considered constructive. All my horrific experiences remained bottled up. I never discussed them nor did I ever seek help. I felt too ashamed, too disgusted and too ugly. Because of this, there was no healthy outlet for all the bad data. It piled up and became etched into my memory. That is how I conditioned myself to deal with the stressors of life. I sucked it up, held back my feelings and kept my mouth shut. I roll differently these days. Now I'm opening up, expressing my feelings and dealing with stress in a way that is helpful. I doubt this will totally erase all bad memory; however, I do believe it will eventually erase the pain.

"Likewise the Spirit also helpeth our infirmities:
for we know not what we should pray for as we ought:
but the Spirit itself maketh intercession for us
with groanings which cannot be uttered."
(Romans 8:26)

Chapter 18

Traumatized

As for me, the tip of the balloon was stretched over life's leaky spigot when my dad left. The dripping was the constant beatings from my brother. This abuse taught me to always be on guard, to be cautious of the clear and present danger that shared my bedroom. In time the valve of that spigot opened wider, causing the slow drip to turn into a steady stream of bad experiences. A predator then opened up a flood of horror.

I met Jay through a Christian outreach during the height of the Jesus movement. Jay took an immediate interest in me. Before long, I was looking up to him as a father-type figure. He drove me to church every Sunday, bought me things and took me to Disneyland and all those other merry and magical places. He also protected me from my older brother. If Rick even looked at me wrong, Jay would tear after him. At six-foot-four and two hundred fifty pounds, Jay served as the ideal bodyguard. I was feeling safe again. Plus, I felt loved.

It wasn't long before I found myself sleeping over at Jay's house on a regular basis. Jay convinced me that he was demon possessed. It wasn't long before these demons began to terrorize the daylights out of me. They were not shy about their intentions either. Their repulsive behavior proved them to be wicked child molesters. When they came to do their dirty deeds, I would cry out to Jesus. Eventually they fled, but not without leaving the smudge of some very foul fingerprints. According to Jay, the demons were the real violators. He claimed he needed me to keep them away and I believed him. I also believed I was safer at Jay's home than at my own. I convinced myself that I could stop Jay and that I could stop the demons, but I could never stop my brother's violent attacks. I also believed that Jay truly cared about me and that he would never do anything to cause harm if he could help it.

Jay was extremely manipulative, using all kinds of creative ways to rob me of my innocence. The abuse and terror continued over the course of a couple years. One particular incident landed me in the emergency room. Back in those days, doctors didn't have an obligation to involve police or social services. I'm very grateful that is no longer the case. Jay should have been arrested. He should have been locked up for what he did. Kids deserve to be protected from predators.

Not for a moment did I ever welcome Jay's perverse behavior. His schemes were never met without protest (or a quick exorcism). Without fail, his touch left me in a most sickened state that consequently kept me that way for prolonged periods. When I finally caught on to his antics, I grew even more disgusted. I also felt stupid, and ashamed. But I never told anybody what had happened, not even my own mother. I never worked these things out with a counselor or minister. I stashed it all. I simply felt too dirty and too foolish to share what went on. I had resolved in my mind that no one would ever understand and that I'd only be regarded as damaged goods.

My only outlet was my pillow. For years I would bawl myself to sleep. I would cry out to God, *"Why? Why me?"* Those tears quickly turned to anger and the anger eventually turned to bitterness. Yes, I was mad! I was mad at Jay for abusing me. I was mad at my father for abandoning me. I was mad at the world and mad at God for every misfortune that had ever happened. Most of all, I was mad at myself for being so foolish. I had a lot of negative energy brewing inside: hurt, pain, self-pity, frustration, unforgiveness and rage. But I didn't talk about it. I kept my mouth shut. And I stewed... for a very long time I stewed and stewed and stewed.

It wasn't until after I turned twenty-two that I came to the end of myself. Unable to carry the anguish any longer, I turned to God and called upon Jesus to save me. What I experienced that day was nothing short of a miracle. All the shame, hurt and anger was lifted in an instant. For the first time in years, I felt free, clean and forgiven. God not only took away my hurt, He healed my heart. I even found forgiveness for those who wronged me. The bitterness was entirely purged, enabling me to move on from the grief.

Though the bitterness was erased from my heart, some bad data was inevitably stored somewhere in the muscle tissue of my pelvis. Furthermore, my childhood trauma had trained my body to always be on guard, especially while in bed. I had been taught well that sleep was a high-risk endeavor. It left me vulnerable. I still remember those nights when I slept over at Jay's house. I would do everything in my power to try and stay awake. Petrified by what might happen, every muscle would clench tighter than a pair of vise grips. The bottom line is that sleeping didn't offer much rest in those days. It wasn't safe - not at home, not anywhere. Warning flags were always sailing. I had no choice but to keep watch.

That was then and this is now. The guard has been dropped. The war is over. Trust has come. The warning flags have been lowered. A banner of love waves in their stead. I feel safe - wonderfully safe. The bed has become my refuge. It's the one and only place in which I feel no pain at all.

Recently, I talked about my abuse for the first time ever. Christy thought it might be helpful on my journey to wellness. She has always been well aware of the fact that I was molested, but I never discussed specifics with her… until recently… after thirty years of marriage. It was painful to recount my horrid past. But wisdom has taught me that it's more painful to bottle things up.

For now, that sad chapter in my life is closed.

The past is the past.

Now I can rest. Even in a bed if I want to.

"And he said, My presence shall go with thee, and I will give thee rest."
(Exodus 33:14)

Chapter 19

Riptide

I spent a ton of time at the beach in my youth. Even before I was old enough to drive, I would find a way to get there from the San Fernando Valley where I grew up. Usually that meant hitching a ride. The Lord be praised, I have no horror stories about hitchhiking, though many people do. As many times as I thumbed my way around, my experiences have all been without incident, but please don't take that as an endorsement. I was fortunate; however, I did encounter danger at my destination on one particular occasion.

The warning flag sailed like a cheery seagull from the Malibu Beach lifeguard station, but I didn't pay any attention to it. The water looked refreshing and the curls were inviting, so I ran in to greet them. I was having a marvelous time catching waves and sitting on top of the world, if that's even possible to achieve without a surfboard. Then it happened. Before I knew it, I was far, far from shore. I attempted to swim back, but only drifted further away. Exhausted by my own efforts, I would wade awhile to catch my breath. In that brief moment, I would be swept out again. Finally, I determined to swim without stopping until my head hit sand. An eternity later, it finally did. When I got up, there was a perturbed-looking lifeguard standing before me. *"You almost drowned!"* he snapped. *"What were you doing out there?"* I felt like screaming at that wise guy, *"Praying for a lifeguard to rescue me!"*

I was caught in what is known as a riptide. They are quite common in the beaches of Southern California. This just happened to be my first encounter with one so severe. A riptide is an undertow below what one ordinarily sees on the surface. The swimming conditions may appear ideal but there is a hidden current that can present a real danger, especially for those who lack the appropriate skills to navigate their way to safety. Such was the case with me. My initial approach was to swim, pause, swim, pause, swim, pause, and, well, you catch my drift. And that is exactly what happened. Each time I paused, I drifted further from the shore. For every stroke forward it was ten strokes back. The moral of the story is: when it comes to riptides, one cannot afford to be idle. You must continually move forward or you will only be taken back further.

Pain is much like a riptide. The best way to overcome it is by moving forward. This is true with regard to both emotional and physical pain. Obviously, I have a load of unpleasant baggage from my childhood. Many of us do. But we don't do ourselves any favors by parking in the past. Nothing good will come of it. Parking in the past will only stir the deadly undercurrent and cause chaos on the surface. It will sour one's countenance, ruin his disposition, poison his attitude and weaken his usefulness as a uniquely gifted human being, one that was created to enjoy a fulfilling and fruitful life.

Parking in the past also takes its toll on one's physical body, causing aches, pain, fatigue, sleeping disorders and a host of other problems. Those who park in the past tend to view themselves as perpetual victims. But much of their suffering is self-inflicted. The fact is that no one has to be a long-term victim. The road to victory is open and accessible to all, but one must be willing to take a step forward. Furthermore, one must also be willing to continue in that direction.

I'm reminded of a line I heard on a movie recently: "Misery is easy, happiness requires effort." No doubt, pain can make one miserable. And to rise above it requires a huge amount of effort. There is both footwork and brainwork involved. Without such things, there is no moving forward. Our riptide illustration applies well here. To go with the flow of an undercurrent requires no effort at all. However, swimming for shore involves legwork and a determined mind. You must forget what's behind and maintain a forward focus. It's exactly as the Apostle Paul wrote:

> *"Brethren, I count not myself to have apprehended: but this one thing I do, forgetting those things which are behind, and reaching forth unto those things which are before."* (Philippians 3:13)

If you have ever seen the Disney classic 'Lion King' you may remember that scene where tiny Timon clobbers unsuspecting Simba over the head. *"Hey! What did you do that for?"* Simba whimpered. *"It doesn't matter,"* the mischievous meerkat replied, *"It's in the past!"* We can learn a lot from that comical cartoon creature. Sometimes we can spend way too much time asking why bad things happen to us. We may never figure out why. It doesn't matter. Move on.

The same principle applies to those who suffer chronic illness and pain. We must move on. We must never allow ourselves to get caught up in the riptide of self-pity. Nor should we ever obsess over the "why" when God is silent. Throughout the entire *Book of Job*, the main characters are bent on getting to the bottom of why Job had to suffer. It was counterproductive and only contributed to Job's frustration. All this nonsense also kindled the Lord's anger. Thankfully, the story ends on a high note - with Job moving on. He quit worrying about the "why" and prayed for those who troubled him. Once he made that step, the Lord healed him and doubled his blessings.

Honestly, I don't know why I was born in a prosperous nation while others end up in some forlorn, third world country. I don't know why some kids are pampered with affection while others fall victim to abuse. I don't know why so many saints suffer while countless sinners are having a ball. Life is filled with unanswered questions. If we understood all the whys, we might be disappointed by the answers. It's best to focus on what we do know. As for me, I know I must move forward.

Spinning my wheels in the 'world of why' doesn't help me - or anybody else.

Here is another thing I'm sure of: if I incessantly focus on my pain, it's only going to get worse. If I make myself worse, I will have more to overcome in order to feel better. Pouting and complaining only set me back further. I open myself up to an ugly riptide of disaster: my pain intensifies, the healing process takes longer and I grow more and more discouraged. Admittedly, I do have weak moments where I fall into this pitiful trap. But once I find myself there, I get out as quickly as possible. I'm determined not to be a victim. I refuse to come out on the losing end of the battle. My best recourse is to move forward and focus on something more positive than my own problems.

Fellow sufferer, we don't have many options before us. As best as I can count, there are two: forward or backward. There is no in-between. We either sink or we swim. We ride the surf above or surrender to the riptide below. Move forward, my friend. Keep your head above water. Catch the wave that flows to the shore of victory and you'll be sitting on top of the world! Once there, the why question will have been answered. You will see the person you have blossomed into and it will all make sense. Until such time, His grace is sufficient.

"And we know that all things work together
for good to them that love God, to them
who are the called according to his
purpose."
(Romans 8:28)

"So the Lord blessed the latter end of Job more than his beginning."
(Job 42:12a)

Chapter 20

You're Being Watched

Recently my daughter, Carly, asked if I was upset with God. I told her I wasn't. She said that she was. She doesn't think it's fair that I suffer, especially in light of my service to the Lord. I assured Carly that God is using my pain for good, that he is growing me, building my faith, deepening my prayer life and teaching me to have compassion for others who struggle with similar issues. I truly believe this and it's important that others know it as well, particularly my children. I desire that God would use my sufferings in their lives and in the lives of all my loved ones. I have come to realize that even pain can become a mighty instrument in the hands of God. So I've given Him mine. There are rules when you surrender your pain to God. Below are the *shalt nots*.

I.   Thou shalt not pout.
II.   Thou shalt not grumble.
III.   Thou shalt not wear a long face.
IV.   Thou shalt not dwell in the past.
V.   Thou shalt never assume the posture of a victim.

What these rules suggest is that for the Lord to use our pain we must repent of all negative thought, speech and behavior. A positive and upbeat attitude is absolutely essential. We must also maintain a hopeful outlook. Furthermore, God uses pain in unimaginable ways when we praise Him in the midst of it.

Fellow sufferer, we have a unique opportunity before us. Nothing testifies to the reality of God like faith in the pressure-cooker of life. The world does not look in wonder upon those who cruise "easy street." Nor do they see much evidence of an Almighty presence there. The road marked with suffering is where the footsteps of the Father are best traced. If, by chance, you travel this road, please be mindful of the many "looky loos" watching on. One day these curious rubberneckers may venture from the curbside and join us. They, too, will journey the road marked with suffering. And they will need the same hope that gets us through. They will need to walk with the One we walk with. Allow them to see Him in your life. Show these curious ones that you are trusting God from start to finish. Should you be serious about this endeavor, you'll need a few more rules under your belt. Below are the *thou shalts*:

VI.   Thou shalt be strong and courageous.
VII.   Thou shalt persevere.
VIII. Thou shalt endure hardship.
IX.   Thou shalt pray without ceasing.
X.   Thou shalt be joyful

Don't ever lose hope, precious one. Never give up on the Lord. He loves you and He will be faithful to strengthen you. He will use you in unimaginable ways to inspire the many looky-loos in your life. Remember, they are constantly watching. Don't lose them. Lead the way. And never forget the rules!

In closing, I'd like to share a letter Carly wrote not long ago. I trust you will find her words encouraging. I sure did. She has stood in the shadows of the "looky-loos." When it comes to suffering, she has walked in my shoes as well.

> *Dear Daddy,*
>
> *I think about and pray constantly for your physical pain. I try endlessly to come to terms with the fact that you do not deserve it, yet God allows it. I also consider my constant struggle with anxiety, but mostly my obsessive thinking that is, in its own right, quite painful. I mourn for you and the physical and emotional pain you must go through each day, yet I am also able to empathize on a small scale how lonely your inner turmoil might be – because how can you explain something you do not understand yourself? And no one can feel physically the agonizing pain you must feel courageously every day. Your inner struggles are what I cling to – they are my testimony that God is real, God is good, God is faithful. Your strength, faith and endurance are a testament of*

God's love, mercy and grace. Not only does your immense pain not debilitate you, but also you thrive! God has not only blessed you in your loyalty, but He has blessed your family, church and the hundreds of broken people you are able to comfort! Because you suffer, you know how to minister to a flock in pain. Thank you for taking such good care of everyone God has ever placed under you, even me. I love you so much and I am always so proud of you.

You are my sunshine,

Carly

*   *   *

"For unto you it is given in the behalf of Christ, not only to believe on him, but also to suffer for his sake."
(Philippians 1:9)

Chapter 21

ThreePartHarmony

If you trust the creation account in Genesis as I do, you know that God reserved the sixth day for His grand finale. That's when He gathered a little dust to make that very first human. Then, from this willing fellow's rib, God designed the perfect partner for him. Each day leading up to that point, the good Lord was merely setting the stage for the main characters, Adam and Eve as well as their many descendants to follow. Now, should you examine the account closely, you will observe a discussion of sorts prior to the creation of our first father. God said, *"Let us make man in our image, after our likeness."* (Genesis 1:26) Notice the use of plurals in that statement: *us* and *our*. Just whom was He talking to, His shadow perhaps? Logic tells us this was a dialogue among the Trinity: God the Father, God the Son and God the Holy Spirit. Each agreed that man should resemble his Creator.

The question must be asked - in what way are we like God? Does this mean that if we were to see Him, it would be as looking into a mirror? Does he have facial features like ours, or a body like ours complete with arms, legs and ribs on the side? Could He easily get lost in a crowd because He looks so much like every other person on the street? What does it mean to be created in His likeness? I believe Genesis 1:26 holds the key. The answer is in the 'us' and 'our'. Like God, we also have a triune nature: body, soul and spirit.

As you ponder this, consider what sets each person of the Trinity apart as unique. God manifests Himself in bodily form through the person of Jesus Christ. God also presents Himself through the agency of the Holy Spirit. Finally, there is the very soul (or nature) of God: His attributes, emotions and personality. In this way, we are very much like Him. Each of us is wonderfully and fearfully designed with a physical body, a soul and a spirit. We truly are three-dimensional, aren't we? Perhaps more than we ever realized!

There is no need to explain the physical aspect of our being. We can observe it with our eyes. The spirit and the soul, however, are another matter. Because each is invisible, they are often misunderstood. I won't get into all the particulars, but for the purposes of our discussion, I should offer at least a brief explanation. The spirit is the part of us that must be born again. It is our spirit that allows us to see the kingdom of God and enjoy an enriching relationship with our Creator.* The

---

* John 3:3

soul, on the other hand, is the essence of who we are as individuals: our emotions, intellect, interests, ambitions, personality traits and so forth. While all these are functions of the mind, they rely heavily on the cooperation of the whole person. The mind, body and spirit must operate in unison, just as the three persons of the Holy Trinity operate in unison. This does not create any challenges for God, but it certainly does for us.

Disharmony among the mind, body and spirit typically results in problems. Each affects the other. When one suffers, all suffer. For example, if I incessantly entertain negative thoughts, it will eventually take a toll on my body. If my spirit is not engaged in the things of God, all will not be well with my soul. If I neglect my body, my mind will revolt and vice-versa. The mind, body and spirit are intricately connected. There most be agreement among the three, for they are one. If harmony is disturbed, all are affected.

The secret to coping and to wellness is to get the mind, body and spirit all in sync. We must also identify what upsets harmony between the three. For example, to undo *what* has happened to my body, I must ask *how* it happened. My pain is not the result of an accident or injury. There is nothing wrong with any of my organs. Nor do I have anything bacterial or cancerous. If a doctor were to examine me (many have) he would find nothing out of the ordinary, at least on the surface. So why do I hurt? And how did I get here? For so long, I had no answers. Now I do. Something disrupted the harmony between my mind and body. In an attempt to purge bad memories from my head, I flushed everything downstairs to my pelvic floor. Over the decades, the trauma continued to pile. That's how I taught myself to deal with bad baggage; I kept a storage room in the basement.

My story is not so unique. There are many physical ailments associated with the mind. Depression is known to wear the body down. Mental stress is a major cause of neck, back and muscle aches, not to mention ulcers. Overworking the mind can cause syndromes such as Epstein Barr, draining the body of every ounce of energy needed simply to rise out of bed. Constant negative thinking weakens the body's immune system. It works the other way as well. There are also things we can do to the body that will impair the mind. If I tank on carbs and sugar, my brain will sign-off before the day is over. If I don't hydrate myself regularly, my head will get lost in a funk. Even as the body fights pain, it can be a major drain on one mentally.

When it comes to the mind, body and spirit, you can't neglect one in order to take care of the other. Attention must be given to all three. There must be a positive flow through the whole person. Our wellness depends on it. There must be inner harmony in order to lead healthy lives. Even our spirits play a huge role in our wellness. When the spirit is satisfied, joy spreads to the soul. If the spirit is neglected, one's ability to cope with hardship and suffering will be greatly hindered.

In a discussion of this nature, one must be especially careful. It causes the antennae of the pagan patrol to go haywire. No doubt, there is a great deal of eastern thought on 'wholeness.' New Agers have a lot to say on the subject, as well. That's not where I'm coming from or where I'm headed. For the record, I am a Bible believing, born again Christian. This chapter is not an endorsement of any of the mystical mumbo-jumbo that's out there. My objective is to reinforce what the Bible has taught from the beginning – that man has a tri-fold nature and that care must be given to the whole person if we are to lead healthy and productive lives.

It is my firm conviction that Christians who lived in the ancient world understood this to a higher degree than we do today. Modern society offers a lot of quick fixes or, more accurately, temporary relief that does little to address the overall health of an individual. So long as we can pop a pill to take the pain away, we don't need to worry about proper diet or exercise or abstaining from harmful vices. As a result, we remain attached to the problem and only pamper its symptoms. Added to this sorry cycle are a host of health experts who praise the power of the pill and do little to promote balanced living. We can't fault them entirely. The tri-fold nature of man is forbidden territory when it comes to the practice of modern medicine. As a result, we have become a pill popping people - whether pills are needed or not.

What does the Bible say about all this? Depending on the translation you read, you will find expressions like "witchcraft" or "sorcery" in several instances. The term used in the original New Testament is 'pharmakeia' from which the word 'pharmaceutical' was derived. So, if you're asking me which remedy is New Age: what I'm proposing or what modern medicine is selling? Frankly, I'm basing my convictions on the Word of God.

By no means am I suggesting that pharmaceuticals offer no benefit in today's world; however I will say this: they are not always needed. And they certainly aren't a substitute for personal healthcare. It is a grave mistake to grow dependant upon pills if the mind, body and spirit are not in agreement or if one or the other suffers neglect. I am proposing that the whole self be cared for. Let's purge our minds of all things negative and fuel them with positive thoughts and uplifting conversation. Let's pamper our bodies with nutritious foods, exercise, rest and recreation. Finally, allow the love of God to pour in and out of your spirit. Nurture it with prayer, scripture reading and the fellowship of other like-minded people. I'm thus promoting a balanced lifestyle that's conducive to wholeness and wellness. Sadly for some, that's too big of a pill to swallow.

*"And the very God of peace sanctify you wholly; and I pray God your whole **spirit** and **soul** and **body** be preserved blameless unto the coming of our Lord Jesus Christ."*

(1 Thessalonians 5:23)

Chapter 22

Am I crazy?

My sincere desire is that this book would offer hope for those who may have lost it. Words could never express how desperate I had felt in the early years of my infirmity, visiting one specialist after the next, seeking some sort of diagnosis. I had undergone all kinds of exams and procedures, only to leave a string of perplexed practitioners scratching their befuddled noggins. All they could offer was an educated guess, which only led to false hopes, further disappointments and a flurry of expenses. It seems *Advil* was a ready recommendation from many experts who couldn't figure me out. Clearly, they didn't appreciate the level of my pain. Advil offered no help at all. Thanks, Doc.

I began to wonder if these specialists all thought I was crazy. Certainly, they had their fair share of hypochondriacs and attention mongers. Did they think I was one because the latest medical journal was silent about me? If all the procedures came back negative did that mean the "nut" test proved positive? Eventually, I gave up on health professionals. Not that I thought they were all bad. They just didn't have answers for my rare condition and I didn't want to be dismissed as a loon. For years I was hopeless. I felt like the woman with the hemorrhage who sought out Jesus:

> *"And a certain woman, which had an issue of blood twelve years, and had suffered many things of many physicians, and had spent all that she had, and was nothing bettered, but rather grew worse, when she had heard of Jesus, came in the press behind, and touched his garment. For she said, if I may touch but his clothes, I shall be whole."* (Mark 5:25-28)

Boy, can I relate! Perhaps you can too. Perhaps you are one who suffered many things from many physicians, spending everything you had on a cure. And instead of being healed, your condition only grew worse. How can that not make one feel hopeless? It did me! I was stuck with a nagging pain that never let up. Furthermore, I was made to feel like a total whack-job. "Take an Advil and have a nice day!" *What? Are you kidding?* Advil isn't too expensive, nor is it a bad thing to have around the house for those minor aches that are explainable, but my pain was major and fell in the category of inexplicable.

Pray-tell me, how is it that remedies like Advil are prescribed for unspecified conditions? There is a pill even for ailments deemed a complete mystery? One doesn't need to understand the problem to know the solution? Is this science or some kind of silly joke? It didn't make any sense to me. I don't know if this makes me smarter or dumber than the experts who sent me on my merry way to Walgreen's. One of us is crazy. I'm sure if you ask them, it must be me.

I am not bitter. I am merely expressing how I had felt at the time, and how numerous others may feel after they've seen countless doctors, undergone countless procedures and exhausted their entire life savings. It's hard not to develop a complex when you're frantic for answers (and a long line of experts look at you strangely and offer some broad wastepaper basket diagnosis). It not only destroys one's hopes, it deflates one's spirits. Those of us with chronic pain and illness are desperate for hope. When our condition is written off as a medical mystery, it does make us wonder if we are taken seriously. It's among the "many things of many physicians we suffer." Before long, we quit reaching for the white coats and start reaching for the garment of Jesus.

I have reached for that garment many times. On every occasion, the answer was the same. As in the case of the apostle Paul, I was led to rest in the sufficiency of God's grace. Though I have yet to receive a physical healing, God has used my condition to bring a greater healing to my spirit and soul, which are of much more value than the flesh. If it takes pain to draw me closer to my Creator, it's a price I'm willing to pay. I'll take His hand over an Advil any day of the week. And it will be Jesus I call in the morning.

Chapter 23

Rest

When the proverbial balloon finally popped, it exploded in my pelvis like dynamite. For weeks, the pain was absolutely excruciating before it finally leveled off to what I now know as baseline. The time leading up to the initial explosion was a long series of hardships, headaches and heartbreaks. This is not to say I was a miserable fellow; I have always tried to maintain a positive and upbeat attitude. But there were huge stressors flooding from the spigot of life into my already stretched balloon. I wouldn't even know where to begin to recount them. To do so chronologically would be impossible. These tragic events dovetailed like mad over a stretch of a couple years, and the memories of them all seem to overlap.

Make no mistake; ministry is not for the timid. The opposition is fierce, the attacks are real and the disappointments are plenty. I watched my own pastor engage in battle after battle, thinking his situation to be unique, or maybe even provoked. Being the nice guy I was, it was certain that everybody would grow to love me. Yes, I would be the lucky pastor of a problem-free fellowship. My rude awakening came early. My sweet disposition didn't stop a certain leader from his inappropriate behavior toward those of the opposite sex. Among other indiscretions, he was ultimately stepped down after pursuing one of our women leaders. She was also married. This man didn't take his demotion well. He grew increasingly envious of his replacement and resentful of me for enlisting a less skilled servant. It wasn't long before he went on a mad campaign to ruin the ministry by spreading a succession of horrendous rumors. Though his lies were quickly exposed, his betrayal left me and many others deeply wounded.

Another dear friend and assistant was also stepped down after being bit by the bitter bug. He wanted to be brought on full-time status, but funds didn't allow it. There were also signs of struggles on the home front with his wife. I kindly explained why the time wasn't right, but he took the news rather hard. With his marriage deteriorating, not being on the church payroll was the least of his troubles. His wife slipped further back into her old lifestyle, met someone else and left her happy home. A few months later, the man she ran off with shot her dead. It was a devastating blow to all of us. She was beloved by many and is missed by all.

During this time, I also got pulled into one of those Hatfield and McCoy type battles. It began with a young couple I counseled not to marry. He was barely nineteen; she was a young mom in her twenties with a four-year-old son. Because this couple had proven to be incompatible and extremely combustible, I thought it best they wait before tying the knot. They saw things differently. With the backing of family, they were hitched at the courthouse. It took only a few months before this new and inexperienced dad attempted to discipline his stepson, leaving some nasty welts on the boy's backside. I was asked by the grandparents to intervene by reporting this incident to the police. I couldn't understand why they, nor the child's mom, made the call. A minister's responsibility is to report *parents* who don't report abuse, not to report abuses for them.

It became all-out war and I was stuck in the crossfire between the numerous relatives who attended our church. The husband's family was angry because I didn't do enough to defend him. The wife's family fumed because I didn't involve authorities. It wasn't long before both families bailed, leaving behind a trail of broken hearts in the wake of their fury. It's always painful when people you care about storm out of your life. You wonder why things end so bitterly when they really don't have to. You long to work things through but are denied the opportunity. It leaves a gaping hole in your heart.

As if we weren't facing enough struggles, our church was in the midst of a building project. This led to one battle after the next with the city and there were a host of financial challenge's to meet their never-ending demands. This not only put a tremendous strain on our small fellowship, but it also put a huge strain on me personally. And with the build-out of our new facility, I was working round the clock non-stop.

It was a difficult season and we got clobbered with one thing after the next. Adding to our list of woes, my in-laws moved from California to be near us. Soon after they arrived, my father-in-law was diagnosed with cancer. It wasn't long before he passed away. My wife was left to care for her mom, who was barely surviving on a respirator. It wasn't long before she passed too. These are just a few examples of what my family was dealing with. It was a trying time not only for us, but also for those we were called to minister to. We felt their pain and they surely felt ours.

I don't want to give any false impressions. There were countless good things happening in the midst of these battles. In spite of all the drama, ministry was happening and the church was flourishing. Unfortunately, I was too busy putting out fires to fully appreciate how God was blessing our fellowship. There were struggles on every front. I finally came to a place where I had no more fight left in me. I grew totally exhausted. I was also depleted of any further vision for our church. I knew I had to do something quickly, something that would bring healing to my heart and restoration to my soul. So, I arranged a trip to Sudan.

Sudan was my Moses moment. It became my 'tabernacle of meeting' where God spoke to me as a friend. As He did with Moses, He promised me: *"My presence shall go with thee, and I will give thee rest."* (Exodus 33:14)

What exactly did God mean when He promised Moses rest? Would Moses be put on light duty? Would the wilderness magically transform into a spa-style resort with water slides and therapeutic hot springs? Would all those whiney wanderers have a freaky Friday with Mother Teresa and others like her? Would they give up their grumbling and all their wicked and rebellious ways? If you know the story, circumstances didn't change for Moses. All those same stressors continued to exist. The wilderness didn't change, nor did all those grumpy people. What exactly did change? *Moses!* He found rest for his soul. He didn't find that in his worldly surroundings, my friend. Note it well: he found it in the presence of God.

Similarly, circumstances didn't change when I returned from Sudan. God didn't pull the plug on my struggles, nor did the devil take a sabbatical. There were plenty of battles to fight and a trail of fires to put out. In short, life, with all its many challenges, marched on. Adding to my many trials, a nagging pain was introduced to my pelvis. In spite of these troubles, there was at least one positive change. I had found rest in the only place I know to find it – in the very presence of God.

Rest is vital to healing. It is also essential for maintaining long-term wellness. Man does as well without rest as he does without food or water. Survival is impossible without it. That is simply how the good Lord designed us. He not only designed us to rest, but

He also commands that we do so. Being the loving Father He is, He understands the consequences we face if we don't.

We need both physical rest and rest for our souls. Should we deprive ourselves of either, the consequences can be absolutely devastating. Lack of rest opens the door for further stress. This perpetuates a vicious cycle, as stress is the chief robber of rest. Rather than put out the welcome mat for stress, we really ought to kick it to the curb. It is rest we should roll out the red carpet for. We ought to run after it like a long lost lover. It sets our entire beings at peace: mind, body and spirit. Stress and rest must be viewed as two opposing rivals. One must be chosen over the other. Rest is the beloved whereas stress is the harlot. Rest is the true and faithful. Stress merely wants to strip and rob you blind. We all have flings with stress, but we must end those affairs quickly. We must surrender to the sweet embrace of rest.

Stress is much too heavy to haul around. It is a bulky and bothersome weight. Stress will tax every part of your being. It will take you down if you let it. It leaves you wounded from the inside out. Stress is the villain you carry and eventually crumble under. On the other hand, rest is something that carries you! It gives you space and room to breathe. It allows you to rejuvenate. It erases the furrowed brow and permits you to smile.

God makes no demands that we should carry any burdens whatsoever. He invites us to hand each and every stressor over to Him. In exchange, He promises rest. When the body is tired, I recommend a soft mattress to lie upon. Should you need rest for the soul, lean upon the Beloved. You will not find rest for the inner person anywhere else. The world only has stress upon stress to offer. It's a mistake to seek rest there. Look no further than the presence of God. Even if all hell breaks loose, in Him there is always rest. Yes, rest upon rest.

"Come unto me, all ye that labour and are heavy laden, and I will give you rest. Take my yoke upon you, and learn of me; for I am meek and lowly in heart: and ye shall find rest unto your souls. For my yoke is easy, and my burden is light."
(Matthew 11:28-30)

Chapter 24

The Point of the Thorn

"And lest I should be exalted above measure through the abundance of the revelations, there was given to me a thorn in the flesh, the messenger of Satan to buffet me, lest I should be exalted above measure."
(2 Corinthians 12:7)

Most have heard of Paul's thorn, but what do we really know about it? There are many speculations about what the apostle may have suffered. I tend to believe it was something of a physical nature as it was "in the flesh." I'm also of the conviction it was a source of nagging pain, as most thorns are. This would also explain why Paul was so desperate to have that poker removed. Perhaps he suffered an injury from a stoning or beating. Who really knows? All we can do is guess. No one can really say with certainty what ailed Paul. For whatever reason, he kept his thorn under a tight lid. He never shared what it was or where he might have hurt. All he offered was why. He states the reason twice: *lest I should be exalted above measure.*

It appears that the Lord didn't want others to make too much of the infamous apostle. People do seem to prop up God's anointed, especially those with popular ministries. Certainly Paul was a celebrated figure in his day. In spite of how all the stuffy religious folk felt, Paul had risen to prominence as leader of the world's fastest growing movement. Lest he be idolized, the thorn served as a steady reminder that God uses ordinary people. To be sure, Paul's thorn also prevented his own head from swelling up like that of a rock star. Scripture does attest to his humble nature. The way I see it, we have the thorn to thank for that.

Paul knew better than to blame God for his thorn. He accused Satan of sticking it to him. Paul graciously conceded that the Lord allowed the thorn, and for a good reason. The Lord intended for Paul to stick it right back at Satan. This is why God allows thorns in your life and in mine. He wants us to stick it back to the one who sticks it to us. The way we do that is by allowing God to use those thorns for good. If God doesn't use them, the devil surely will. Ultimately, the choice is ours. Fortunately, Paul looked to the Lord in his season of suffering. And let us never forget how blessed the church is because he did. That's the whole point of the thorn.

Thorns become like crosses in a way. Neither one is anything anybody would ever ask for. Because they are associated with pain, we ask for them to be removed. Paul did three times. Jesus prayed a similar prayer in the Garden of Gethsemane. As the cross drew closer He prayed three times, *"If it be possible, let this cup pass from me."* In the same breath He uttered, *"nevertheless not as I will, but as thou wilt."* For God to accomplish His good purpose, there was no getting around the cross. It just wasn't possible. And though the cross was painful, it produced a world of good for all of us.

Similarly, it was after the third prayer that Paul quickly realized he was stuck with the dreaded thorn. God assured Paul that he was stuck with His abounding grace as well. Seeing firsthand all the good produced as a result of God's grace, Paul declared, *"Most gladly therefore will I rather glory in my infirmities, that the power of Christ may rest upon me."* (2 Corinthians 12:9b) Though the thorn was painful, God used it powerfully in Paul's life to accomplish a mighty work.

I'll admit I'm no Paul, but I do desire that God would use my thorn to accomplish a world of good. Should you find yourself stuck with a thorn, you would benefit from making that your desire as well. Firstly, you must accept that God wants to accomplish a great work in your own life. He is more interested in our character than our comfort. And sometimes He needs to cause some discomfort in order to build our character! For Paul, the issue was pride. God used that rascally thorn to keep him humble. Now, that may not be God's purpose for your thorn. Perhaps he wants to develop you into a more compassionate person. It could be He wants your prayer life to deepen. Maybe He wants to stretch your faith a little. Or maybe He just wants you

---

* Matthew 26:39

to lean on Him more. The possibilities are endless. The important thing is that you remain open and teachable to whatever it is God is trying to show you.

Once you allow God to use that thorn in your own life, He will surely use it in the lives of countless others. But do you see why you must first allow the Lord to do a work in you? Unless that happens, the thorn will only be a source of misery, and it won't be of any value to anyone else. It is your response to the thorn that determines how it will be used, or who gets to use it – God or Satan. Once you hand that nasty thorn over to the Lord, great things will happen. You begin to marvel at what God is doing in your life. You marvel at how God uses you to touch the hearts of others. That's when you can glory in your infirmity as Paul did. That right there is a powerful testimony. When pain turns to praise, people listen. It inspires them like nothing else can.

I don't know how long I will have my thorn. It could be a few months. It could be years. But for however long I'm afflicted with it, I want God to use it. I want God to be glorified by it. Therefore, I've dedicated my thorn to Him. I guess were both stuck with it - at least for a while.

Chapter 25

Carwash

I generally don't have meltdowns, but I did yesterday. I was having one of my not-so-good days. If I might be so bold, it would even rank as a really bad day, at least pain wise. My problem is, I don't want pain to tell me what I can and cannot do. Too often it is a mean and unfair dictator. So, when asked by my daughter, Birdie, to drive with her to the new *Mr. Clean Carwash* across town, I rebelled against that harsh voice deep inside and agreed to go. Sometimes I just can't be deprived of life's simple pleasures. Being a dad would be one of those.

If you didn't catch on before, I will state again: sitting is not my best position. Now, when it comes to car seats, they are oftentimes unbearable. It only took a few minutes of being strapped into Birdie's Jeep Cherokee before my pain shot through the roof. Determined not to spoil our time together, I bit the bullet as best as I could to conceal my agony. That said, however, I probably wasn't the most chipper company to have around. My mind was elsewhere - fighting a losing battle - so words with Birdie were few.

By the time we arrived at *Mr. Clean's*, I had no choice but to bail out. I confessed to Birdie my predicament and quickly leaped out the door like a wounded animal. Making my way inside the waiting area, I watched my daughter's old Cherokee plow through a gauntlet of suds. Blinded by the multitude of spinning brushes, she never noticed me, nor did she see me wave as she floated by as if in slow motion. I wanted Birdie to know I was right there with her, but she was enraptured into a heavenly world of foam. I realize that driving through a carwash isn't anything spectacular. Anybody with a dirty, old jalopy and a few bucks can enjoy the experience. But this was a moment I wanted to share with someone extremely special in my life.

My pain only worsened on the drive home. Gritting my teeth the entire time, I again said very little. Upon our return, I bolted into the house, ran to my bedroom and buried my face into my pillow, soaking it like a sponge with streams of hot tears.

I had not wept like this for as long as I can remember. I wept for many reasons. I wept because I could not enjoy a simple outing with my daughter. I wept because Christy and I had a dinner engagement with friends that evening, and I knew we would have to cancel. I wept because I was the cause of too many other cancellations. I wept because I probably wouldn't be able to make the drive to see my granddaughter dressed in her Halloween costume the next day. I wept over every simple pleasure that pain had stolen from me. I wept because my condition had gone on for too long. I desperately wanted to be well again.

Christy eventually found me blubbering on my soggy pillow and quickly came to comfort me. She felt bad for the pain I was in and grieved because she didn't know the right words to say. I'm not sure there really are any right words. It's just nice to have someone there who genuinely cares and understands the tears of a grown man. That goes a lot further than being told everything will turn out fine. Hurting people need compassion, not an endless succession of greeting card clichés and false hopes.

My dear wife assured me it was okay to cry, that it was even necessary. At the risk of sounding self-absorbed, it was even deserved. The alternative would have been to bottle up more hurts, which is how I got to where I am in the first place. Perhaps the tears are an indication of growth. I'm finally learning to let my emotions come out in a healthier way. I must admit, crying did do me a world of wonders. I felt much better afterward. The tears comforted me like a warm blanket.

Shortly after my little meltdown, Birdie paid me a visit. I told her how badly I felt about the situation and how desperately I wanted to do "dad" things with her unhindered. I assured her that I would be well one day. I never want her to lose that hope either. We hugged and told each other, "I love you."

Later, Christy took Birdie out for sushi. I spent the evening relaxing in a hot bathtub listening to Etta James on *Pandora*. There were no candles lit. There was no wine poured. I had poured enough tears to soothe my sorrows. I had treated my Lord to another fresh bottle.

"Thou tellest my wanderings: put thou my tears into thy bottle:
are they not in thy book?"
(Psalm 56:8)

Chapter 26

High Hopes

I've only known a couple people who suffer the same condition I have. One of them is Randall. He attends *Calvary Austin,* where I serve as pastor. Randall has gone through great extremes to get well. He put up a wad of money for surgery. Rather than relieve him of his agony, the procedure only added to it. Randall's surgeon told him that it would take time for him to notice any difference. It's been several months now and the only difference he really notices is that his pain is more severe. One can only imagine his disappointment.

I opened an email from Roger this morning. I'd like to share it with you.

> *"Had a rough day today with my pain. It was bad enough I couldn't eat dinner. It just takes over. I am praying for a new perspective on it. I think I'm at that place where I've just learned to live with it and not get my hopes up. Maybe that means I've lost hope of healing and I know that's not what God would want me to think. You are very encouraging in your messages and even your blurbs on*

'Facebook.' I wish I had that. I've been praying for a new perspective and I can only be changed by God Himself.

When I am doing pretty bad I do think of you and it reminds me go pray for you. How is your therapy going?

In Christ
Randall

Admittedly, I do feel a lot like Randall at times. Especially on those really bad days, I wonder if I'll ever be healed. After months of therapy, I struggle to discern God's will in this matter. Do I keep hoping? Or am I better off I accepting my pain as something I'm stuck with for the long haul? Should I choose the route of acceptance once again? Would that be the same as hanging it up on hope? Or would it help me to move on and gain a healthier perspective on reality? Hope is a good thing, but false hope only leads to heartbreak. We all know this, but we can't always discern one from the other.

Last night, I contemplated these thoughts while lying awake in the wee hours. That's why I was quite surprised to find Randall's email when I rolled out of the sack. Sometimes it's a tough call knowing whether to accept an illness or to hope for a healing. The path of hope is not shy of hurdles, even when hope is genuine. There is always the temptation to quit, do nothing or fumble into another direction. And in the desperate world of the chronically ill, those options pop up like weeds. They make hope difficult to hold onto. They create doubt and cause questions. They boast of easy outs but deny their dead ends. And, Lord knows, there are zillions of hucksters on the Internet promising quick relief for a price. These vultures aren't stupid. They know people will pay anything if they are desperate enough; those with chronic pain generally are.

With regard to my own condition, I have resolved to continue with the stretching and relaxation exercises prescribed to me. Though this regiment has yet to reduce my pain level, it has been beneficial in countless other ways. Honestly, I have never felt healthier. And from everything I have heard and read about my unique infirmity, my exercise program is the only shot I have at getting well, even if it takes years. The other thing that has been drilled into my head is – don't lose hope. So I continue to do the possible and trust God for the impossible, even if His sense of urgency seems to trail behind mine.

Randall's email also served as a ready reminder that people do watch me – people who desperately long for hope. That is the message I wish to impart to you, fellow sufferer. There is a world of hurting people out there who are seeking hope. May it be that they could look to you! When we feel hopeless, we give others permission to feel that way too, and that is not what this world needs. Now, hope does not mean that there is a pot of gold at the end of every rainbow. Nor does it mean everybody gets a supernatural healing if they wave the name of Jesus like a magic wand. Hope simply puts us at rest in the loving arms of God. It reminds us that His grace is sufficient and that we can do all things through Jesus Christ who strengthens us. By the way, Paul meant he could cope with any hardship when he made that claim. (See Philippians 4:12-14)

Perhaps you are one who must accept your condition as permanent. This does not mean you ought to give up on hope. It does not mean you ought to roll over and waste away as if you had nothing to live for. It means that in spite of the pain, you are to move forward and trust God to see you through another day. With this comes the unrelenting conviction that God wants the ultimate best for you. The world needs this kind of hope more than well wishes. Sufferers look to other sufferers wondering, "How do they get through life? What is their secret?" You may not have the power to heal the hurting, but you certainly have the ability to help them. You can show them that chronic illness is not meant to kill the soul. You can prove that one's spirit can rise above any pain. I need this kind of encouragement on those especially rough days. Don't we all?

While we're on the subject, I should probably define what the biblical meaning of hope is. When we say hope, it can mean a variety of things. Often, we use the word *hope* to describe wishful thinking. When a person says, "I hope to win the lottery!" he fully realizes that odds don't swing in his favor. There will be no surprises (or disappointments) if it doesn't happen. It's not really expected to happen, at least in the mind of the rational thinker.

The New Testament term for hope is 'elpis' in the original. It is the Greek expression for 'expectation.' For example, I fully expect to go to heaven. I don't spend my days wondering if I really will. It's not like the lottery where all odds are against me. I have the assurance of God's promise. Therefore, I fully expect the pearly gates to open wide upon my arrival. There are no worries. When it comes to my pain, this is the kind of hope I cling to. I fully expect God to use it in my life and also in the lives of others. I fully expect God to see me through each and every day, no matter how terrible things get. I fully expect to see God glorified in my suffering. That's what biblical hope is. That's the hope the good Lord wants for all of us. This is the kind of hope our world desperately needs. We are not put on this planet to spread wishful thinking. We are here to help others have reasonable expectations. To be used of God is one of them. To get through the day is another. This is what keeps spirits high and frees us from all worry.

"According to my earnest expectation and my hope, that in nothing I shall be ashamed, but that with all boldness, as always, so now also Christ shall be magnified in my body, whether it be by life, or by death." (Philippians 1:20)

"And hope maketh not ashamed; because the love of God is shed abroad in our hearts by the Holy Ghost which is given unto us." (Romans 5:5)

Chapter 27

Once Upon a Plane

Pastor Nick is another fellow I know that suffers from CPPS. He serves as pastor of a prominent church in Siegen, Germany. Years ago, when we were both in better shape, I ministered alongside of him as a youth pastor. My big concern about moving to Germany was the weather. Siegen is in the northern part and it gets freezing cold up there. Prior to this big move, I battled upper-back pain for many years. The worst flare-ups occurred when temperatures dropped below the forty-degree range. Living in Southern California, that didn't happen all too often. In Siegen it happens a lot. But that did not deter my family and I from going. The amazing thing is – for the entire two years we lived in Germany I never had any back problems, nor have I had any since. I do believe in miracles. I'm living proof that God is able to heal, should He choose to do so.

Recently, my wife and I returned to Germany to speak at a retreat for Nick and his flock. It had been thirteen years since we had been back. Having an advance notice of almost ten months, I was certain that I would be fully rehabilitated before taking this long journey. With my particular health condition, sitting in an airplane passenger seat for an extended period is not a grand idea. I can barely handle an hour of sitting on my best day. But God had healed me before! And because I was headed in the very same direction as my previous healing, surely an encore wasn't out of the question.

God had other plans. The big miracle is that I survived the flight. It was absolute murder and there was little I could do to find one ounce of relief. I didn't have a hot bath to sink into. I didn't have a soft mattress to plop onto. Every so often I could stand, but for the most part I was confined to a miserable seat. Seriously, it was like torture, hour upon hour of sheer torture. Were I a hostage being forced to cough up top-secret information, I would have sung like a bird.

I cannot begin to tell you how relieved I was to get off of that plane. Nor can words adequately express how much I did not look forward to the four-hour drive to the retreat center. At least when traveling by auto, one can stop, get out and stretch a little. Thankfully, these frequent road trip breaks were guaranteed, as our trusty driver Nick needed them as much as I did. That is one benefit of traveling with someone who also suffers from CPPS. The thing is that you don't meet people with this condition every day.

There does seem to be a kindred spirit that exists between fellow sufferers, which I cannot fully explain. I suppose it's like other groups that are pulled together by a common thread. Musicians, for example, seem to get each other in ways that are beyond me. They can bond for hours and discuss things that those outside their peculiar world are clueless of. We who suffer chronic illness and pain also find ourselves in a peculiar world, and within it there is sweet fellowship to be found. It is a community built on mutual understanding and compassion. We have the unique advantage of identifying with one another. "I feel your pain" is something we say and truly mean. Many people don't understand the world I now live in. They don't fully grasp what I deal with day-to-day. Nick does. And I get him. I feel his pain.

God had a purpose for me in Germany. He also had a purpose for not healing me while being there. I was able to encourage Nick in his sufferings, and he was able to encourage me in mine. It was a pivotal moment for both of us. I had answers to our condition that he was searching for. This enabled him to seek further help and he is more hopeful as a result. Nick was also a tremendous encouragement to me, affirming my usefulness as God's servant to others who hurt. This gives me great hope. All and all, it was a fulfilling week for the both of us as we smothered each other in comfort and prayers. I had no idea this was part of God's plan, but I left Germany with that sense of 'mission accomplished.'

You're probably wondering about my flight home. It wasn't comfortable, but it wasn't too painful, either. There was enough discomfort to remind me that I wasn't yet healed. But there was just enough relief to assure me of God's mercies. Perhaps you have to be part of that strange world of the chronic sufferer to understand this, but we receive these moments as gifts from above. By the time I got off that flight, I praised the Lord for His all-sufficient grace.

"Therefore my heart is glad, and my glory rejoiceth: my flesh also shall rest in hope." (Psalm 16:9)

Chapter 28

God Calling

"But the God of all grace, who hath called us unto his
eternal glory by Christ Jesus, after that ye have suffered
a while, make you perfect, stablish, strengthen, settle
you."
(1 Peter 5:10)

There are important principles to consider when battling a chronic condition. They are outlined in the above verse, so take time to chew on it for a good while. Allow each word to churn in you mind and descend into the depths of your heart. Let them settle into your innermost being. Hopefully, what I share will only confirm what the Spirit has already revealed to you.

Peter speaks as one who is well acquainted with suffering. Obviously, his words are inspired from above, but we also hear the voice of wisdom, born from firsthand experience no doubt. Peter's statement is chock-full of helpful insights and heavenly hope, all neatly packaged in a solitary sentence. I pray you get out of it as much as I did.

The first thing we must understand is that with suffering comes a high and holy calling. There is an expectation that we answer that call; however, we are never pressured to do so. The choice is totally ours to make. But you need to know something. Answering the call holds all the perks, whereas *not* answering offers zip. Now, should you accept this mission, it is vital that you know Him who calls - the God of all grace! This means He will grant you the grace to endure whatever degree of suffering He allows.

One must also understand the extent of God's calling. He calls us unto His eternal glory. In other words, He is not willing that our sufferings be wasted. He sees them as remarkably useful. Ponder this for a moment - nothing has impacted history more than God manifesting His glory through suffering. By the same token - nothing has impacted *eternity* more than God manifesting His glory through suffering. The Lord will also work wonders through your sufferings if you let Him. He will change you as well as the countless others around you. The legacy you leave may even impact generations to come. Furthermore, you will behold God's glory like never imagined.

It's important that we see the big picture and recognize how God desires to use human suffering as a means of manifesting His eternal glory to a needy world. And let us never lose sight of how He wants to use suffering in each of our own lives as well. He truly does care for the sufferer and has big plans to bless us. That's the good news, along with this: our suffering is only for a while. We don't take it into eternity. Only the glory it produces remains. For this reason the Apostle Paul boasted:

> *"For I reckon that the sufferings of this*
> *present time are not worthy to be*
> *compared with the glory which shall be*
> *revealed in us."* (Romans 8:18)

The future glory is what we have to look forward to in the hereafter; however, Peter reminds us that God also uses our sufferings here and now. The Lord seeks to improve our lives in four crucial areas: He longs to perfect us, establish us, strengthen us and settle us (after we have suffered a while). Let's analyze these four areas and find out exactly what God is after.

God plans to perfect us!

Though that may sound far too ambitious, it's true. But "perfect" may not mean what you think it does. I hope you don't have the idea that God allows us to suffer until we are free of every last flaw. We'd all be in serious trouble if that were the case. For a clearer understanding, here are some definitions of 'perfect' from select Bible concordances: complete, mend, equip, put in order, adjust, strengthen and, finally, "make one what he ought to be."[*] The last definition sums things up rather nicely – God wants us to be all that we can be! Unfortunately, there are no shortcuts and the process can be rather painful at times. Just as with surgery, before one can fully mend, he must endure the

---

[*] Strong's Concordance

pokes and jabs. Yet He who began the good work will be faithful to complete it. (See Philippians 1:6)

God plans to establish us!

I once had the privilege of planting a church in San Marcos, Texas. It took time before this fellowship could rightly be considered "established." There was a lot of blood, sweat and tears poured along the way. As any church planter will tell you, getting things off the ground can be a pain-staking process. One must endure seasons of suffering and uncertainty. In the end, though, the pay-off is huge. In my case, I had the honor of seeing a budding fellowship develop into a healthy, vibrant and well-established church body.

I share this experience to illustrate how God works within us. Nothing gets established simply by existing. There is work involved, painful work. God could just turn us loose like wind-up toys and watch what happens, but that is not His way. He wants to build us into something strong, healthy and vibrant. He wants to establish us as fully functional, purpose driven people with something positive to contribute to society. Shaping us requires work. Plenty of blood, sweat and tears can be expected. However, the pay-off is huge, should we endure. We will be much more useful beings and have a better understanding of our place in the world. With this comes great contentment.

> *"Now our Lord Jesus Christ himself,*
> *and God, even our Father, which hath*
> *loved us, and hath given us everlasting*

consolation and good hope through
grace, Comfort your hearts, and stablish
you in every good word and work."
(2 Thessalonians 2:16-17)

God plans to strengthen us!

If you have ever worked out at a fitness club, then you are familiar with the old saying, "No pain - no gain." Getting into shape is never easy. Just to stay in shape can be a real pain! If only we could get the same results without sweating or suffering. Unfortunately, such isn't the case. Building a body is agonizing, and so is trimming the fat. The same is true when it comes to strengthening the soul. Character building is painful, as is shedding the flesh. But the end result is always the same – we come out much healthier should we hang in there. Spiritually speaking, all of us have some beefing up to do. We all have dead weight that needs to go. God allows us time in the 'world gym' to improve our condition. He seeks to make us fit and strong. He knows we'll feel better once we're in top shape.

God plans to settle us!

Most of us prefer to be comfortable. That's why we resist change. We don't want anything to interfere with our cushy norm; however, if change doesn't happen, we run the risk of growing stagnant in life. We never reach our full potential and simply coast along like lost corks in the storm drain. It usually takes something radical to purge us from a complacent existence. It might be a job change. You advance from a mediocre position to a highly paid one. Perhaps relocation is involved - from a small rental in the city to beachfront property. The transition can be frustrating, but, ultimately, you know you're moving on to a better place. Eventually, you will settle and enter into even greater blessings.

That's how it is in the journey of life. God has not called us to a mediocre existence. He wants us to reach our full potential. As He draws us out from our comfort zones, the transition is often painful. Yet in our hearts, we know He is leading us to a much better place. He settles us somewhere nearer to Him. We need to remember that in our seasons of suffering. We are merely in a state of transition. God is moving us to someplace special. Hang in there. Don't settle for anything less.

Chapter 29

Dung Beetles!

I can't imagine a life any lower than that of the Dung Beetle. These poor creatures spend a lot of time with poop - elephant poop to be precise. They roll the stuff into huge balls four times their size then use it as a nesting place (where more cute dung beetles hatch and are introduced into the pile). Once the offspring come to a ripe age, they too will carry on the foul tradition of pushing poop. Like those that go before them, they embrace a lowly life in Dumbo droppings.

I am extremely grateful that God did not call us to this kind of existence; however, there are those who settle for one like it. All they see is the poopy side of life. Because they are so focused on the putrid pile before them, they fail to see the splendor on the other side This is an easy snare to fall into when you're dealing with pain on a continual basis. It's hard not to focus on it. And the more you do, the more it stinks. It becomes like a huge wad of waste that must constantly be pushed around. One can easily grow weary and lose perspective on all that is pleasant. That's when the glimmer at the end of the proverbial tunnel eclipses to black. The light is still there, you just can't see beyond the waste.

No doubt you have heard the saying, "when life hands you a lemon, make lemonade." My message is similar: *Get your eyes off the poop pile. Look up*! It is impossible to cope with pain without a positive outlook and an upbeat attitude. We must accept that sometimes there is no getting around Bandini[*] Mountain, but don't pitch your tent there. Keep pushing ahead until you make it to the other side. In the meantime, keep an upward focus! Life tends to stink when you fixate on the smelly stuff.

Perhaps you were also taught to, "Count your many blessings. Name them on by one." That seemed to make sense back when we were kids. Then, as we grow older, we start counting our many bummers and naming them one by one. This can develop into a bad habit if we're not careful. It's also a sure path to depression. If you haven't seen the studies, depression typically goes hand-in-hand with chronic pain. This is why it is not uncommon for antidepressants to be prescribed as part of the treatment. It doesn't take a genius to figure out that physical pain is a real downer. In light of this fact, I make it a point to have a celebration service in my devotion time each morning. There is no better way to begin the day. It sets me off on the right foot without fail.

Prayer time can easily turn into one miserable pity party when the bulk of it is spent crying, *"Woe is me."* I strongly advise against that. It only sets the stage for a

---

[*] A major fertilizer brand. Bandini Mountain is a metaphor and not an actual place.

lousy day. It's okay to ask for a healing. I also do that every now and then. But it's not a healthy place to park. I strongly urge that you devote more of yourself to praise and thanksgiving. It really does help one get out from under that stinky ball I've been talking about.

I like to divide my praise into two parts. First, I thank God for all the heavenly blessings. Secondly, I thank him for all my earthly blessings, with the understanding that every good and perfect gift comes from Him. encourage you to do the same.

Under the heading of heavenly blessings, take time to thank the Lord for things such as: His love, salvation, forgiveness, the cross, the Word, the Holy Spirit, mercy, grace, etc. Should you ever draw a blank, read carefully through the first three chapters of Ephesian and highlight all those wonderful perks you have in Christ. You can use this as a ready thanksgiving list. And it's okay to peek at it when you pray! Just make sure you're sincere and not rattling things off as if you were knocking out a checklist. That's when prayer is reduced to a monotonous religious routine, and religion won't make you feel any better.

Under the category of earthly blessings, be thankful for such things as: family, friends, the roof over your head, the food in your pantry, the clothes on your back and the very air you breathe. Obviously, those are but a few examples. I suggest that you compile a more extensive list. Once again, the good Lord won't mind if you peek at it now and then, so long as you are truly expressing thanks from your heart.

Also be sure to thank God for answered prayer! Thank Him for what He has done, what He is doing and what He has promised to do. Make a habit of praise. Develop an attitude of gratitude. It will truly improve your outlook. It will help you cope better with your pain and with life in general. In addition to making yourself joyful, you will also make God really happy. He inhabits the praises of His people and blesses those who offer it.

"The Lord is my strength and my shield; my heart trusted in him, and I am helped: therefore my heart greatly rejoiceth; and with my song will I praise him." (Psalm 28:7)

"Why art thou cast down, O my soul? And why art thou disquieted within me? Hope in God: for I shall yet praise him, who is the health of my countenance, and my God." (Psalm 43:5)

Chapter 30

Never Cry Uncle

Chronic pain does have a way of working itself to the top shelf in every bad situation. It behaves like the codependent mistress who refuses to play second fiddle. When other difficulties arise, pain will not relent from that number one position. She slaps and screams, demanding your full respect. Whatever hardship is added to the mix, pain won't be ignored. She grows even more unruly. You can't forsake her to deal with the next issue. She's the boisterous companion to every other problem that comes along: pain plus financial problems; pain plus family problems, pain plus problems on the job and so on. She is the ever-present elephant in the room. There might be a hundred other things sharing the same space, but it's that giant beast that stands out most. And the only thing celebrating her presence is the icky dung beetle beneath her stinky tail.

What I want to say here is this: if we don't get a handle on this pain thing, the other burdens of life will surely clobber us. I know. It happened to me.

After three years or so, pain finally robbed me of all my zest. I just didn't know how to function anymore and, as a result, my ministry quietly slipped into cruise control. Things were getting done, but it was the same ol' same ol'. I knew I had to do something to stimulate new life - both in me and in the church body entrusted to me. I thought that establishing a new work in the neighboring community might be the perfect jumpstart. So, I met with my faithful leaders and discussed a Saturday evening satellite service, to which I was given a rapid-fire, thumbs-up salute. Everyone was in agreement without exception.

Apparently, one leader was more zealous than I realized and sought to start his own work in the same community. Unbeknownst to me, he secretly shared his plans with other congregants and paved the way for a painful church split. I never saw it coming. This particular leader and I had been friends for over ten years and never did I suspect he was capable of instigating a division, let alone betraying me. We had always gotten along extremely well. I can't even recall a time we ever had one cross word. There were no arguments, squabbles or disagreements preceding his devious plight. All I can assume is that I had something he wanted and he sought to possess it.

My poor friend's greed quickly led him down a sad and sordid path of underhanded behavior. To sway others his direction, he promised the moon and filled people's ears with propaganda designed to discredit me. Before I knew it, those once cherished as dear friends were bailing out the door, angry for reasons I was never made privy to. The ripple affects that this split created were tremendous. Many who remained were lost in confusion over the whole ordeal, wondering what I might have done to upset so many people. I had no answers. All I knew was that the rumor mill reaped havoc on our poor church.

Several who left returned after realizing they were merely pawns in a cunning power play; however, my wounded heart was still riddled with feelings of abandonment and betrayal. Not only did I feel discarded by those who left, but I also felt that all trust was lost among the precious saints who remained. Any self-worth I might have had during this time went down the flusher. I was damaged goods as far as I could tell.

The brutal combination of pelvic pain and a broken heart was more than I could bear. I contemplated leaving the ministry once and for all, and sunk into a terrible depression. I was so depressed that my eldest daughter bought me a gift certificate for a Christian counselor. I was so depressed that I actually went! That chivalrous shrink spoke rather frankly, insisting that wasn't cut out for the job of a pastor. He went on to say that I didn't have what it takes to handle the disappointments associated with ministry. Who was I to argue?

It wasn't long after this counseling session that I called a special meeting with our church body. Christy and shared from our hearts how we were wounded by the unexpected exodus, and how every ounce of wind had been sapped from our sails. I was completely honest with our group. I announced that if for any reason I could no longer be trusted, it would be unfair for me to continue as pastor. It was an extremely emotional evening for all of us; there wasn't a single dry eye in the house. Before we knew it, our pity party transformed into an all-out love-fest.

Somehow, my precious wife and I wound up on the receiving end of a massive agape gusher. The support we received was phenomenal. Some wept when apologizing for buying into all the vicious gossip. Others sobbed as they voiced appreciation for our years of service. There were tears and more tears, a keg-full for my Lord. Just between Christy and I, an entire box of Kleenex was emptied.

It was this meeting that helped me realize that the time for leaving was not right. Others besides me were hurting, and with that in mind, abandoning ship was not the loving thing to do. Besides, the church had suffered enough loss. My resignation would only tear the wound deeper. God also made it clear that in order to finish well, I needed to follow Him and not my fragile little feelings. I quickly repented of all self-pity and self-centeredness and chose to rise above my hurts. It was a major turning point for me as well as for our entire congregation. The Lord brought full and immediate restoration, ushering us into a season of unprecedented fruitfulness.

As much as I hate to admit it, church drama is not unusual. The wise shrink was right - pastors must be prepared for an unholy host of disappointments. I wasn't. Looking back, I understand the benefit of this preparation. I was in a bad shape to begin with. Pelvic pain had already locked me into a full nelson, making it easy for a groin-kick from the next attacker. When the eager leader went rogue, I was outnumbered. Pain plus betrayal pinned me into a corner and laid on a chokehold. I have since learned that I must put my pain under submission. Unless I do, the next villain that comes along will have me crying uncle in no time.

Few contend with the struggles of full-time ministry, especially those unique to the role of senior pastor. However, no one gets through this life unscathed. Though your brand may differ from mine, suffering is common to us all. Even Jesus said, *"In the world you will have tribulation."** Therefore, we shouldn't be surprised when troubles come our way. Like it or not, they're to be expected.

For those of us who deal with chronic pain, we must hang tough and rise above those everyday struggles. Unless we do, the next storm that comes along will wipe us out completely. This wipeout is bound to happen should you view yourself as a victim. Speaking from past experience, this is a sorry place to be. Nor is it one anybody should ever settle for. Jesus not only said, *"In the world you will have tribulation,"* but He went on to say, *"But be of good cheer, I have overcome the world."* This tells me that I don't have to cry uncle or give in to my pain. Through Christ Jesus, I can bring

---

* See John 16:33

it under submission. You can as well, so be of good cheer!

Epilogue

It's Thanksgiving Day. I am with family relaxing in a rustic old cabin overlooking the Blanco River just on the outskirts of Wimberley, Texas. Just beyond the sliding glass door, oak trees wave boasting of a perfectly blue sky. The aroma of roasted turkey fills the room, with a hint of sweet potato. Or is it pumpkin? From the next room I hear all kinds of happy chatter and the laughter of one small child, my granddaughter – she was born to entertain. Aside from these welcomed interruptions, all is peaceful. I soak in my surroundings like a beluga-sized sponge. I look, I listen and I smell the flavorful scents of autumn festivities. All this I do from a sitting position. Remarkable indeed!

Last night I sat for a good while. This was not done without discomfort; however, my pain was tolerable. Today, my pain is minimal; it is lower than it has been since I can remember. I believe this chapter of my life is soon coming to a close. I am on my way to wellness. Yes, I will be wonderfully whole again. I will be granted the luxury of sitting whenever I want for however long I wish. And I will enjoy the privilege of sitting as never before. For so long, I took this blessing for granted. Never again! I will thank the Lord each day for allowing me to park my weary bum wherever it may land. My heart will leap with joy whenever I set my wishful eyes upon a chair or stool or a creaky old bench (or even a cold, damp porch step). I will once again partake of simple sitting pleasures like reading, writing or watching out the window on a rainy day.

I am grateful for this painful journey; God has used it in my life for good. The lessons chronicled in this book were all gleaned in the valley of suffering. They have prepared me for the next adventure, whatever that may be. Perhaps I will go to Africa; the missionary spirit in me has grown restless. It will not die. It must be released even if I am not completely healed... even if it kills me. I will go to Uganda, to the city of Kampala. I will share my story as an encouragement to others. The African people will surely be amused. They will chuckle at how trivial my sufferings are compared to theirs. And I will look upon their cheerful faces with thankfulness.

AUTHOR BIO

Terry Michaels has had the privilege of serving in ministry for many years. He worked extensively with youth at *Calvary Chapel San Bernardino* in California and *Calvary Chapel Siegen* in Germany. Terry also served as founding pastor of *Calvary Chapel of the Springs* in San Marcos, Texas and currently pastors at *Calvary Austin*. Terry also has a background in broadcasting. He worked as a radio personality in California area markets such as Palm Springs, San Bernardino/Riverside and Mendocino. He is author of four books. Terry resides with his wife, Christy, in Austin. They have two daughters and a granddaughter.

www.terrymichaels.org

www.calvaryaustin.com

51724584R00079

Made in the USA
Charleston, SC
02 February 2016